# Opening to the Real

# Opening to the Real

Frank R. Sinclair

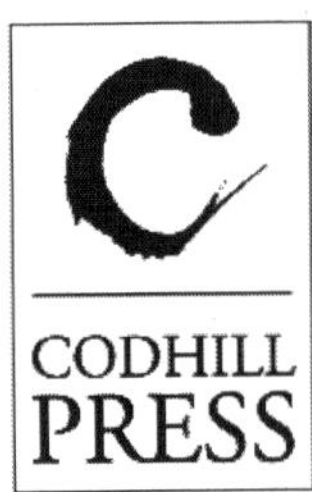


Codhill books are published by
David Appelbaum for Codhill Press

codhill.com

Opening to the Real

 First Edition.

Published in the United States of America

ISBN 978-1-949933-06-2

## Acknowledgements

I would like to thank a number of people who have helped me prepare this book for publication.

I am grateful to Carl Lehmann-Haupt for permission to publish the preface to his book *Martin Benson Speaks*, and to Greg Loy, editor of the *Gurdjieff International Review*, for permission to include the tribute to Beatrice Sinclair that appeared in the review's spring 2018 issue.

I wish to thank Luis Morales for his design and graphics help, and David Myers for his cover design. I wish also to thank Myers and Barbara Dartley for their generosity in transcribing the material that appears in Part II.

Mary C. Arendt, author of the tribute to Beatrice mentioned above, provided invaluable help in preparing the manuscript for publication and tying up loose ends.

Of course, I alone am responsible for the content collected here, the judgements made, and the thoughts so freely expressed.

Frank R. Sinclair
Nyack, NY

# Contents

# Part I

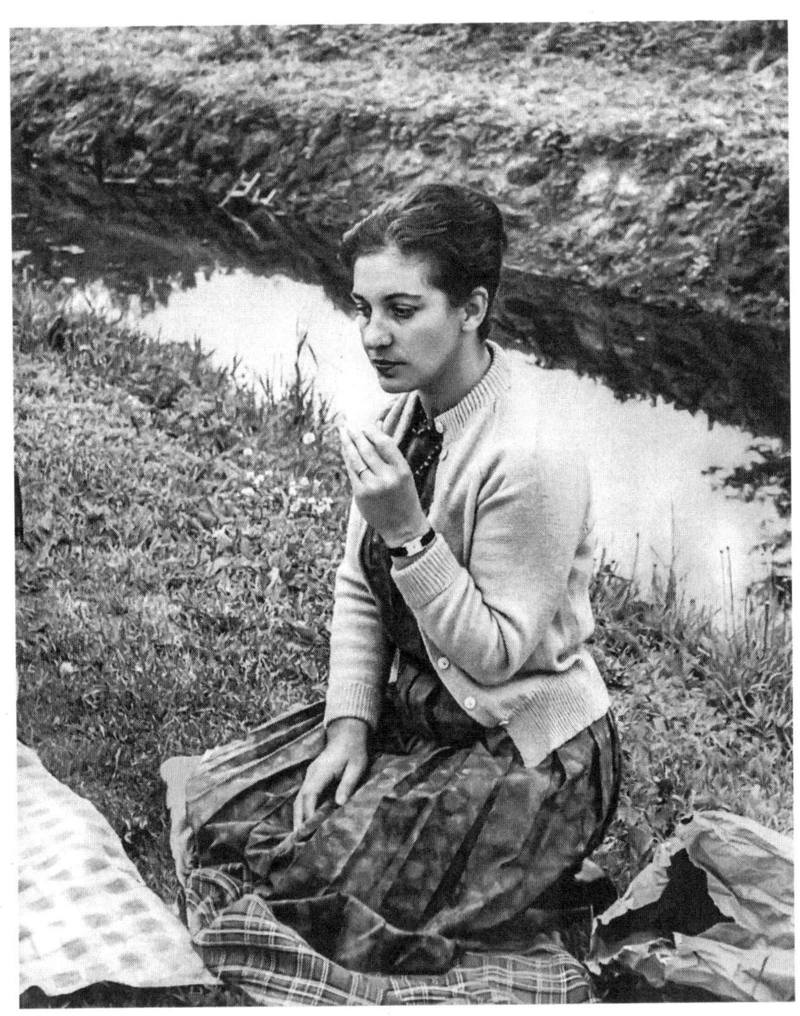

Beatrice Sinclair, around 1960.

# Beatrice Sinclair and the Practice of the Presence of God

I am presenting this little volume of recollections and assessments primarily as a belated yet totally deserved tribute to Beatrice, my wife of forty-nine years.

As readers of this present report know, I had written two rather well-regarded previous books about my involvement with the teachings of G.I. Gurdjieff, which prompted at least one reviewer to wonder why I had not given more information about the woman who had shared my life in the process. So permit me to rectify my evident though unintentional lapse.

Still, in the hasnamussian surroundings in which we find ourselves on our benighted planet these days, the truth is that certain self-appointed commentators almost automatically try to ensure that our tenure is judged to be either well-beloved or penetratingly accursed—by their standards. One's personal mission is indeed to be unencumbered by the gratuitous burden so readily disgorged by these all-knowing entities.

Of course, the overriding observations in this present book are largely confined to reports such as those of the sittings that I conducted in the Gurdjieff Foundation of New York, and therefore carried very little personal information. In looking for "filler" material, I could quite quietly have pointed out how the remorseless tendentiousness on the part of some professedly all-knowing literary entities plays itself out at every level in an organization such as the Gurdjieff Foundation. Indeed, I had more or less playfully planned to write a little chapter titled—and describing—"Chief Features I Have Known" among these all-knowing entities, given that most esoteric (and other) weaknesses are invariably all but unknown and invisible to the actual perpetrators and/or victims themselves.

In my case, these ubiquitous commentators—who, being so removed from any discernible struggle, should properly be unnamed except in a footnote, I suppose—have rather unceremoniously given me short shrift in their otherwise well-meaning assessments of my attempts during the past sixty years to describe my impressions of the Fourth Way.

But Beatrice, who was ten years older than I, had the great privilege that I did not have of actually being in Gurdjieff's presence and sitting at his feet. Indeed, he had told her, "I like your type." Beatrice, in fact, had told me of some extraordinary encounters, including one in which she had witnessed a remarkable shift—truthfully, a transformation—in Gurdjieff's presence: in one moment he had been chastising a talkative woman at one of his dinners, saying, "Your hair color of shit," and then in the next moment it was "as if he was in the very presence of God," Beatrice recalled.

Beatrice served and cherished and respected the Work. She did not try merely to promote her engaging egoism. Back in 1948, as a prize-winning graduate of the Rhode Island School of Design, she was methodically embarking on her career as a schoolteacher, and she loved her role "out there" in life, eventually guiding children for decades in one of the leading schools in New Jersey.

It was in her last years that she devoted herself to the daily inner discipline known as the "practice of the presence of God" as exemplified by the seventeenth-century Brother Lawrence.

And then, in her very last days, when I visited her in hospital to bring her back to her home on the waterfront in Grand View on Hudson, where she hoped to die, she actually exemplified the "seamless departure" that I have been hoping to have for myself. Our old friend and mentor Martin Benson was the model—dying with his eyes wide open. And there in her hospital room, surrounded by a few unbelieving nurses who sensed that she was approaching her end, Beatrice made her astonishing ultimate observation to me: "I am dead. I have died."

The next day, there was some delay in the arrival of the ambulance bringing her back home from the hospital while we set up a bed in the living room. She died just a few minutes after being laid in her bed.

At this point in my narrative, I should commend a nameless literary blogger on some of his references to my declared understandings of the Work—this in spite of his insistence that what he missed in both my books was "a pen-portrait of Beatrice, Frank's companion for almost fifty years." He notes that "She was surely a patient and positive woman in her own right, his helpmeet in the months of his greatest stress." Indeed, he accorded me a rather fanciful literary status by declaring that Sinclair "shares this unwillingness to go into detail with Dante." Dante, no less.

But I should not be carping. He graciously mentions that Beatrice, "who was raised a Roman Catholic, found solace in the writings of Brother Lawrence, a lay brother of the Carmelites in Paris in 1666, whose spiritual handbook bears the provocative title, 'The Practice of the Presence of God.'"

In any event, readers of our blogger's two reviews will probably be intrigued by the discussion of the chapter "John Pentland: The Lordly Line of High Sinclair" in my book *Without Benefit of Clergy*. The point is that neither Lord Pentland (family name: Henry John Sinclair) nor I ever traded on our so-called bloodlines. Indeed, I recall the interesting moment when Lord Pentland came to me while I was washing dishes—yes, management had me washing dishes—in the kitchen at Armonk and asked to speak to me. We went outside, away from any casual eavesdroppers, and he told me that Madame de Salzmann wanted me to be a member of the Armonk Council. I had been her choice, not his.

Nevertheless, I did end up sitting alongside Lord Pentland as a member of Group One at the end of his life. I was also appointed to the presidency of the Foundation by the founding fathers in New York. And for those not in the know, I am proud to say that I worked closely with his wife, Lucy, Lady Pentland, both in the New York Foundation and in several years of visits to the Work in Los Angeles. And I consider their daughter, Mary Rothenberg, as blood of my blood.

But since *Without Benefit of Clergy* has been mentioned—and quietly dismissed by certain all-knowing standard bearers of the truth—I should take the opportunity to thank Jeff Zaleski, editor and publisher of *Parabola* magazine, for his fearless declaration that "This book is a worthy companion for any spiritual seeker, and the most insightful memoir of the Gurdjieff Work published this century." I recommend it for some extraordinary accounts of life out on the edge, as it were—if not the beautiful photograph of myself on the crux pitch of Jacob's Ladder on Table Mountain. In any event, one of these ubiquitous bloggers did concede that my book displayed an "earnest quality of life," for which, I should note, I had quietly sacrificed my family, my country, and my professional career in order to live at Franklin Farms in its final years.

Meanwhile, it was actually rather early on that I was privileged to meet Beatrice's great friend and mentor, Swami Jyotirmayananda, founder and head of the Yoga Research Foundation in Miami, Florida. It all began with the fact that one of Beatrice's sisters, Lee, had a swimming school on the oceanfront in Santurce, Puerto Rico. One year Swami Sivananda passed through Puerto Rico and Lee was so touched that she followed Sivananda back to his ashram in Rishikesh, India. Evidently, Lee—who now went by the name Swami Lalitananda—made no move to return to the U.S., and Beatrice and others were concerned.

So when Madame Olga de Hartmann, widow of Gurdjieff's famous conductor and composer, told Beatrice she was planning a trip to India, Beatrice asked if she would try to learn just what Lalitananda's intentions were.

Madame de Hartmann later reported that she had found Lalitananda living on the outskirts of the ashram under the tutelage of one of Sivananda's leading assistants, Jyotirmayananda. I never learned whether Madame de Hartmann had had any hand in persuading Jyotirmayananda to come to the Americas, but lo and behold, both swamis turned up at Mendham one Sunday, invited by the Russian lady. They made dashing figures in their orange robes at the Sunday lunch discussion, but were not invited to speak. The swami is actually a year younger than I am, but he had a masterly understanding of his mission. As I write, he is still headquartered in Miami.

I was privileged to pay many visits to the two swamis in Miami, and have maintained contact with Swami Jyotirmayananda all these years. I can report how touching it is to read his monthly letter in his magazine, the *International Yoga Guide*, which he addresses to every one of us as "Blessed Self, adorations."

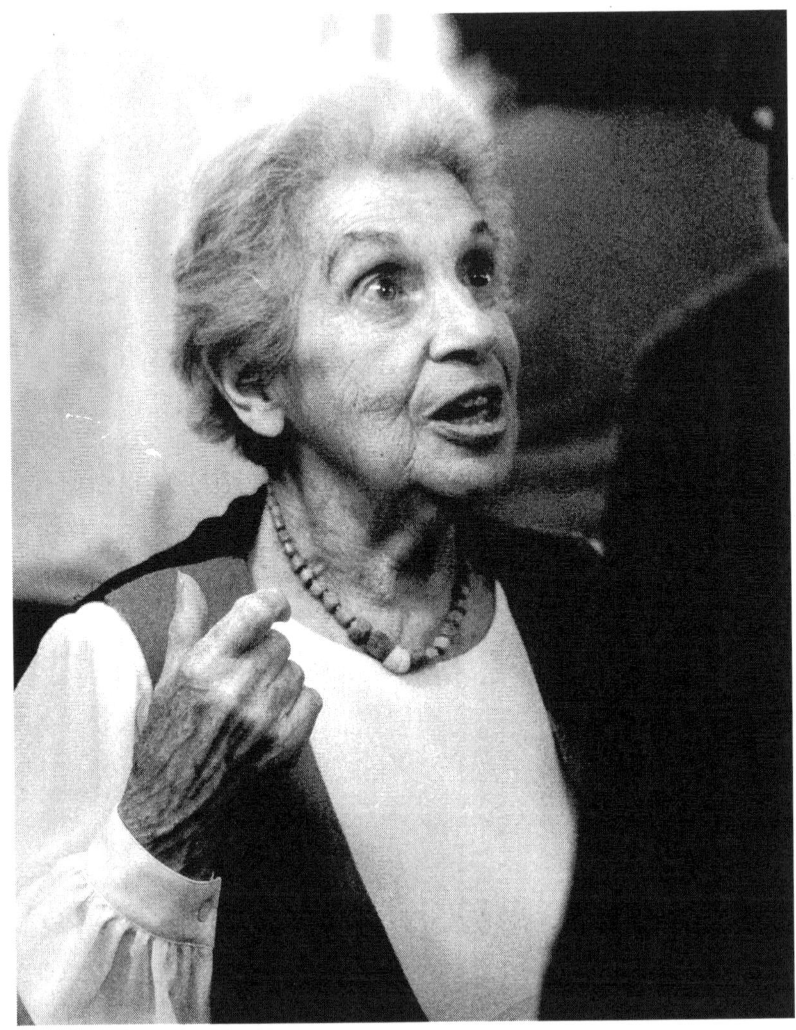

Beatrice was always engaging and positive. G.I. Gurdjieff, whose teaching she cherished and respected, told her, "I like your type." This photo was taken during an exhibition of Beatrice's artwork.

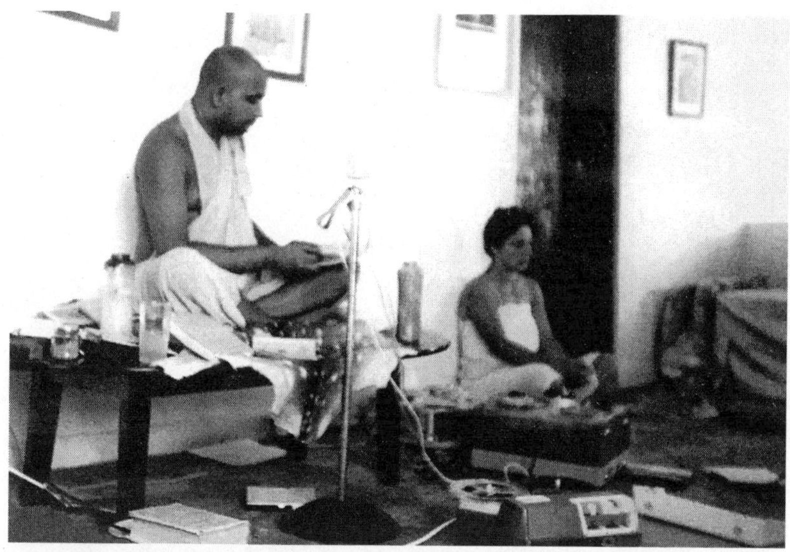

Swami Jyotirmayananda , left, founder and head of the Yoga Research Foundation in Miami, Florida, was a great friend of Beatrice's and her sister Lee (Swami Lalitananda).

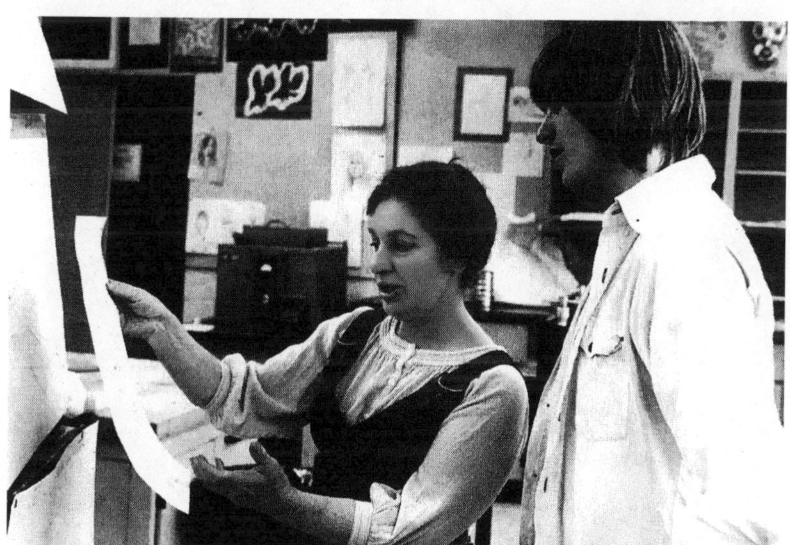

As a schoolteacher, Beatrice guided children for decades in one of the leading high schools in New Jersey. She loved her role "out there" in life.

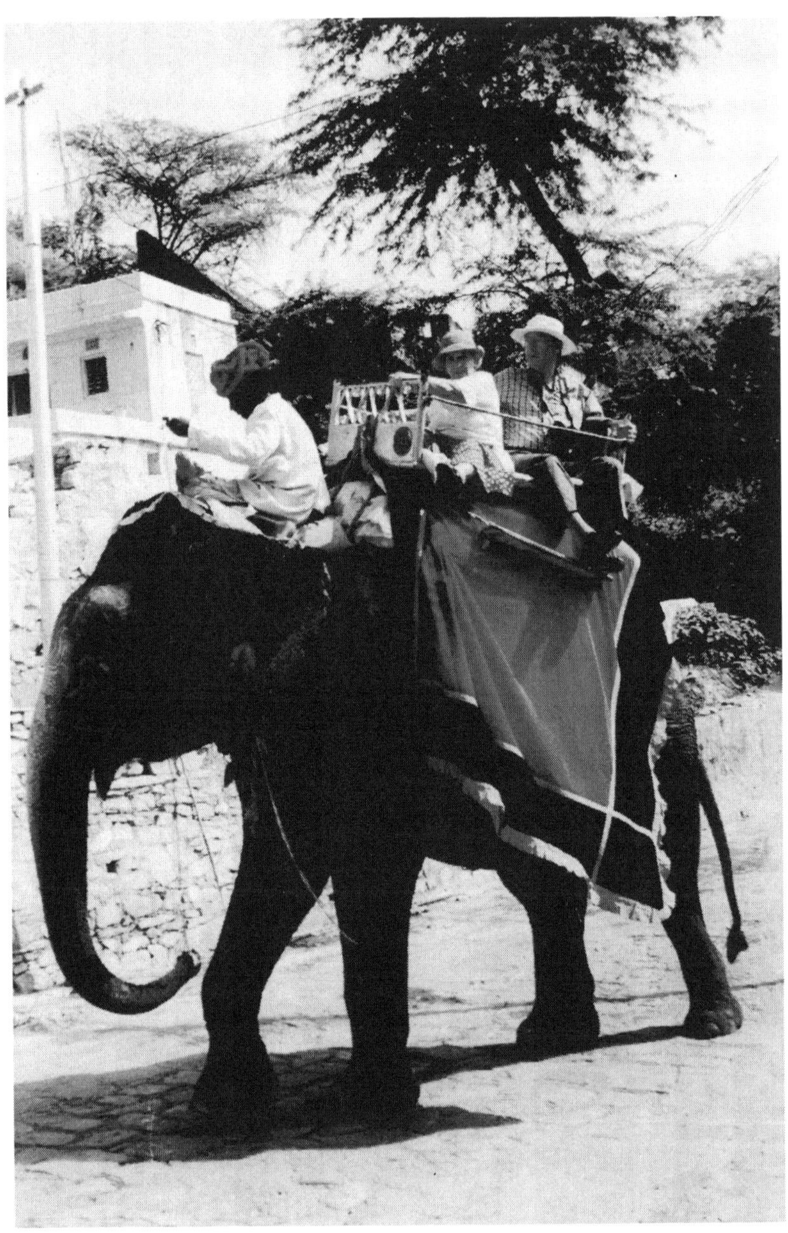

India was among the places that Beatrice and Frank traveled to in later years.

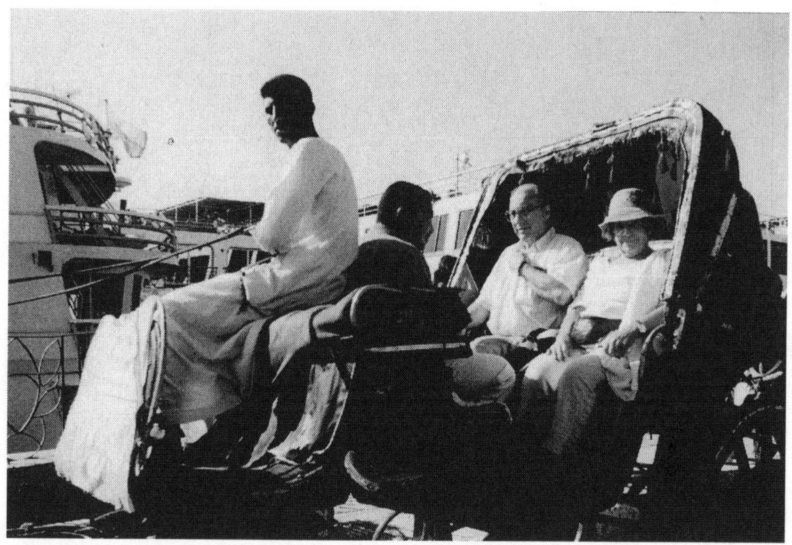

They also traveled to Egypt.

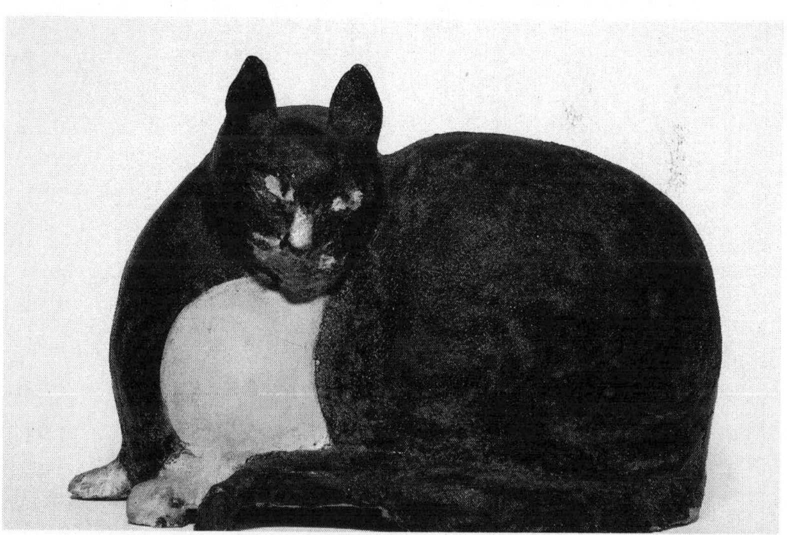

The inspiration for this meditative cat, which Beatrice sculpted later in life, came from a cover of an issue of *Material for Thought* that featured a Chinese painting of a cat.

# "From One Sister to a Brother"

*This is a typed version of a handwritten letter from Lise Etievan, dated Friday, April 21, 2006.*

Dear Frank:

Today it is Queen Elizabeth II's birthday. Early this morning I finished reading your book, "Without Benefit of Clergy" which you sent me about two months ago. As soon as I received it I plunged into it, but couldn't go on being involved, with so many things "to do." I mentioned the publication of your book to Michel Peterfalvi, and even gave it to him. He told me, then, that he was interested to read it, especially concerning Martin Benson with whom he worked on the Chicken House roof, when he went to Mendham, during 3 weeks in summer, not long after Mme Ouspensky's death. But I made sure that Michel would return the book, so that I could finish reading it during the Easter Holidays. They are now over, and I can say that I read every single line of your book. I can also say that at closing it, I felt the impulse to come back to it again and again. Each chapter is so rich, contains so many strong impressions and fine knowledge, that I feel and recognize that I haven't been able to take them in sufficiently. Quite honestly I'll indicate to you my favorite chapters, which I believe will not surprise you:

Chapter 5: "Where is He That is Born?"
This chapter is so full of unbelievable experiences that it helps the reader to understand more about the play of forces. I realize that such shocks can only lead to a completely new approach of what is life, what can take place between people, even in a so to say House of Work. I understand more the process that took place in you when you felt the need, the urge to integrate the inner and outer currents of life. Through the price you paid in your suffering, it led you to be granted to perceive more about a greater reality.

Chapter 6: "Every Nationality has Something I not Like"
What a beautiful picture of Beatrice! There is in this chapter one beautiful sentence: "Everyone felt this level of love—divine love. Perhaps this is why we were able to take so many of his shocks."—Please give to Beatrice my love.

Chapter 12: Jeanne de Salzmann, "A Compelling Call"
After reading this strong chapter, my wish is that it should be as soon as possible translated in[to] French—but I intend to speak to you about it, when we see each other in May in London.

Chapter 13: "Some Random Inferences"
These chapters represent, in various ways, a great help. Mainly they help to reconsider more strongly the need for the state of questioning which is usually so restricted, poor, of opening more our eyes, ears, heart and mind. I have been particularly sensitive and happy innerly because I found in your chapters so many places treating the theme of "Attention," often containing a subtle reference to a hidden dimension, [a] scale of unknown qualities which need to be discovered patiently.

I agree with you, Madame de S. was the only person in the Work who was able to help us to vibrate to this FORCE, to make us feel the importance of it in our inner development, through her own presence. Untiringly she returned to the core of that Search, to this central study. I appreciate the words you report: "A body of Attention." What a call!

As you know I had the luck to be more or less in contact with many mentors in the Work during my ten years in [the] U.S. This luck allows me to follow with interest all of the impressions you related about them, ending each time with a wonderful sense of recognition for the efforts they produced to sustain the "Work," most of them for decades. All of them, at one point or another[,] have been touched by "Another Light" during their existence on the Planet Earth.

Now a few words about my response to your chapter 13. I feel, precisely at this period of time, [that it is] so useful to look at the past of the Work, under a vision of various landscapes. I feel also this necessity—and your active mind helps me—to be able to know more clearly, to embrace what each period brought as possibilities and misunderstanding since Mr. Gurdjieff's death. In front of the impressive changes that took place during several decades[,] I can't help remembering Madame de S.'s strong call, and question she brought, each year (wherever she was), at the moment of resuming our gatherings, our many activities connected with the Work necessities:

"Now, how do you feel and understand the state of the Work?" Each time she was touching an intimate note—feeling the responsibility to let us know the need to look closely in what way we were out of gear. In other words, I felt she was again questioning us:

—Is our search actively turned toward the encounter with a real "I"?

—What do we need to learn now, to abandon now on one side, and in another side to engage more into?

—How to live a sincere movement of returning to the essential, and be at service?

These questions are more or less shared today among the oldest in the Work. When they are shared we feel as if Madame de S. were still with us. Otherwise....

Well, I wrote too many words. But before reaching the bottom of the page, I wish to express to you, Frank, my sincere thanks for all the efforts you put in, to give birth to "Without Benefit of Clergy." I believe it is going to give a strong impact to and among the "Searchers of Truth" in the World.

From one sister to a brother.

Lise

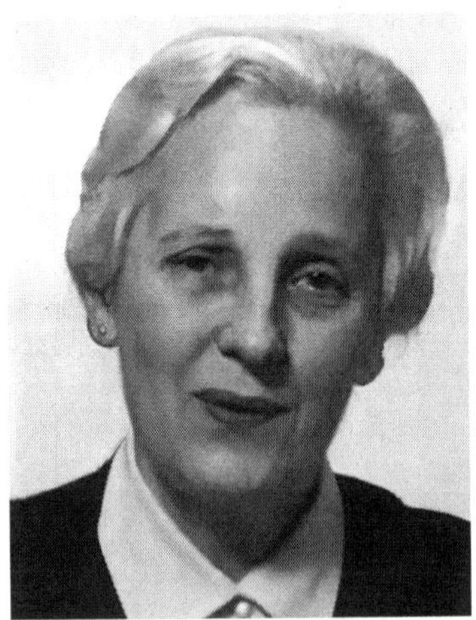

**Lise Etievan**

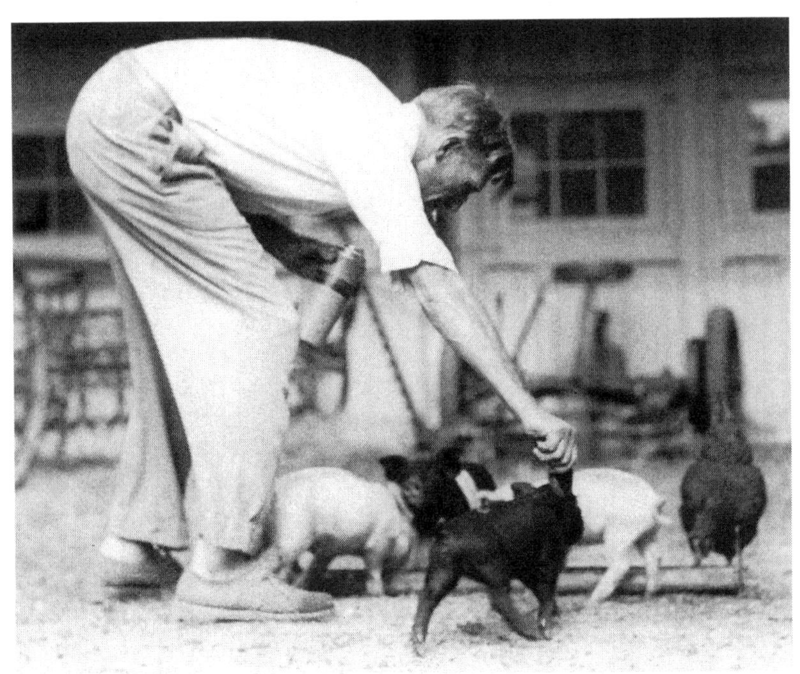

Martin Benson, Franklin Farms, around 1960.

# "Don't Make Logic"

*I wrote this piece on Martin Benson as the foreword to the previously published* Martin Benson Speaks, *edited and with an introduction by Carl Lehmann-Haupt. It is reprinted here with permission.*

The remarkable Greek-Armenian spiritual master and teacher of dancing, G. I. Gurdjieff, drew an extraordinary range of people into his orbit—scientists, musicians, physicians, artists, psychologists, philosophers, to name a few. And not the least among these students was an unusual but true son of the soil, Martin Benson. The fascinating trove of reminiscences and reflections contained in this book reflects something of the depth and originality of Benson's understanding of the work for being as conveyed by Gurdjieff. Now, after being kept under wraps for several decades, it is only fitting that Benson's insights can be shared.

Thanks to Carl Lehmann-Haupt, who taped this material during the last months of Benson's life, a pre-publication reading of some excerpts was presented at the 2011 celebration of Gurdjieff's birthday at the Armenian Cathedral in downtown New York. I introduced this material to the listeners, all members and friends of the Gurdjieff Foundation of New York, by sharing some of my own personal recollections of the time I had spent in his company as a young man. What follows is adapted from that slight introduction.

Benson had been the last gate keeper—and the man who locked the gates for the last time—at the Prieuré, Gurdjieff's estate in Fontainebleau, France, where he had established the Institute for the Harmonious Development of Man. He was later a potent and unorthodox presence at Franklin Farms, the Ouspensky estate in Mendham, New Jersey, during its last few years as a place of Work. And later still he was the presiding spirit in the rather unorthodox ice house at Armonk.

Benson was a man of great simplicity, complexity, and compassion. He had been wounded in action on the Western Front in World War I when hardly out of his teens. Shaken by his experiences, he retreated to the Ramapo Mountains to live among the strange folk of the hills. It was there, as he used to say, that the Work found him, which is a whole untold story in itself.

He was just about to turn 60 when I first encountered him on my arrival at Franklin Farms, in August, 1958. After only a week on the estate, I admitted to Miss Dorothy Darlington, who managed the household that looked after Madame Ouspensky, that I could make neither hide nor hair of what Benson was saying. She assured me that he had indeed spent some time with Gurdjieff, and that Gurdjieff had said of him that he was "more in essence than in personality." This was all very mysterious to me, and I took it as a task to keep an open mind.

For about eighteen months I lived under Benson's wing, as it were, working at his side from the crack of dawn often until well after midnight. In the evening, after I had finished my tasks in the main house, he would have me come to his cottage. And there he sat me down and spoke for hours in the same unstructured and unscripted way that comes through in the pages that follow. It was as if he were wrestling in his whole being to find the words to express his search. If I even so much as nodded, as I occasionally did after the long hard day out on the estate, he would poke me in the chest and say, "You don't do that."

And then there came the day when, with the profound compassion and understanding of a man who had himself known suffering, he would acknowledge my own devastating experience of remorse. "You are one of my people," he said. We never ever spoke about that afterwards. But there was clearly a real bond, because one day when I was quietly raking leaves at his cottage he turned to me and said, "Sinclair, I don't know why you came, but I am glad you came."

Although you could not parse his sentences, as Roger Lipsey once said of him in a beautiful poem, Benson was no simpleton, no unlettered bumpkin. But he was certainly not an intellectual either, not remotely a member of the intelligentsia. "Don't make logic," he used to say. And even though his obituary in *The New York Times* said rather imposingly that he was an "agriculturalist," he had never regarded himself as anything other than a man who tilled the soil, shoveled manure, wielded an axe with purpose and precision, tended horses and cows and sheep and pigs and chickens—and spoke to them and they to him. He was, in his very marrow, a farmer.

I learned, too, that he loved music, from Bach to songs of the Civil War, and he loved to sing. In fact, on a number of occasions while making my rounds at night, I would find him roaming the grounds during thunderstorms, singing in some strange and nameless tongue to the trees and fields and to the heavens, an elemental man breathing in the vibrant life around him.

After Madame Ouspensky's death at the end of 1961, the Foundation acquired an estate in Armonk. I recall how the brash young Turks of that time, who boasted that they were going to usher in a "new" era in the Work in New York, had no place for Benson in their plans. But he staked his claim to a derelict wooden building known as the ice house, where his loyal stalwarts from the Mendham days installed themselves. The ice house was, as our poet expressed it,

> ...a club for heavier men
> Who lumber up the path of consciousness together
> With fair doubts about lighter men elsewhere on the grounds...

It was in the ice house that Benson and his crew demonstrated some novel and free-form building techniques, and converted the old brick baking oven into a forge. They straightened and secured the sagging roof by running a rough-hewn tree trunk horizontally down the middle. He used to tell Madame de Salzmann, "That's the Nigerian—we're spearing its jaw." And it was there that this "club for heavier men" continued Benson's passionate exploration of resonance and sound, and built their famous Aeolian, or wind, harp.

Madame de Salzmann loved the atmosphere of the ice house. After Benson died and his team disbanded, I was allowed to turn the ice house into a print shop, and Madame would come down and just stand to one side watching us at work, not saying anything. Perhaps it was hallowed ground to her as well.

So, now, to hear Benson speak in the rough-hewn way he used to speak. Let the reader brace himself.

# A Being Who Loved Life

By Mary C. Arendt

*This tribute to Beatrice was previously published in the spring 2018 issue of the* Gurdjieff International Review, *when the theme was "Pupils of Gurdjieff." Reprinted here by permission.*

Beatrice Sinclair had a magic about her. She was, in fact, magical. One could not be in her presence for long and not feel the sparkle and joy that hung in the air around her. For me, it was because she loved life, all life, totally.

I was introduced to Beatrice soon after meeting the Gurdjieff Work in New York and joining a group led by her husband, Frank. It was the early 1990s, she was perhaps in her 70s, I was about 30, and the Sinclairs had invited five of us to Easter dinner at their home in Grand-View-on-Hudson. Her height alone, at less than five feet, was intensely captivating. One of the guests, a young male actor, also new to the Work, was somehow persuaded by Beatrice to read aloud from a tale by I think Hans Christian Andersen ("The Story of the Wind"?). The scene made quite an impression—not the tale or hearing it read aloud, but Beatrice herself and the atmosphere of wonder and wise innocence that both enveloped her and that she radiated as the story unfolded and she sat, literally, on the edge of her seat.

The following November, this same small group of mainly younger people joined Beatrice and Frank for Thanksgiving (I was a long way from my family in California), and soon, as I became more immersed in the Work ideas and less interested in the pursuits that had marked my 20s, I was visiting regularly, usually on Sundays and mostly in the warmer months. On these Sundays I would help Beatrice in her pottery studio or, more often, in the garden. We sometimes took her car (whose interior was a kind of automobile equivalent of Gurdjieff's famous pantry) and drove to the local nursery. These were wonderful outings, providing me with an education in basic horticulture and the chance for conversation with Beatrice. While I drove, she might ask me about literature (I had majored in English at Berkeley) or to recite lines of poetry, such as these from Gerard Manley Hopkins: "The world is charged with the grandeur of God" and "Glory be to God for dappled things." There was also, one of my favorites, William Carlos Williams's spare "The Red Wheel Barrow," which for both of us captured how the everyday and our relationship to it could suddenly be imbued with a transcendent quality ("so much depends / upon / a red wheel / barrow / glazed with rain / water / beside the white / chickens").

Anyone who saw Beatrice at her home on the river could feel her extraordinary sensitivity to things of the earth—to flowers, trees, birds, and other animals, especially baby animals—and to beauty. Beatrice was sensitive to life, and she had a remarkable ability to awaken that sensitivity in others. Krishnamurti, whose talks she often read or listened to, and whose photo she had pinned up near her papers and books, said something that I think really captures this quality that Beatrice had in abundance. He said: "To be sensitive is to feel for people, for birds, for flowers, for trees—not because they are yours, but just because you are awake to the extraordinary beauty of things." Beatrice was awake to beauty. And not, I think, because she was an artist—though she was that, and a very fine, very grounded one whose inspiration came mostly from nature. Beatrice was awake to beauty because, unlike so many of us, she was not encumbered by the need to prove herself. This meant she was free to see, really see, into the heart of whatever was before her—an object, a plant, a bird, a face, a picture—and discern its specialness. She could take the most ordinary thing—a print advertisement for Apple computers featuring a photo of the Dalai Lama, for example—and elevate it to something profound simply by placing it—carefully, attentively, just so—amid her surroundings. Her enclosed, sun-filled porch at her home on the Hudson was filled to overflowing with postcards of paintings, sculptures, and icons; photos of animals and nature torn from newspapers and magazines; black-and-white photos of people like Krishnamurti; and quotations from books copied out in her modest script—all lovingly positioned. Beatrice knew what she liked, and she liked to be surrounded by beautiful forms, harmonious colors, and meaningful representations.

To quote Krishamurti again: "[T]he moment you have in your heart this extraordinary thing called love and feel the depth, the delight, the ecstasy, of it, you will discover that for you the world is transformed." Anyone who had the good fortune to visit Beatrice on her porch or in her garden could see that she had this love, because when you entered her world you experienced a world that was different from the one you saw. Her world had a shine; it sparkled and was somehow blessed. What I found so extraordinary was that in looking at the world through her eyes, I could feel how generous she was, and kind, and absolutely without an agenda. This aspect of her nature—which as she got older seemed only to intensify—had a way of causing those who dared to put themselves above her to reveal the opposite in themselves, their disingenuousness and lack of generosity. She was without guile. It's no wonder she got along so well with children. They grew wide-eyed in her presence. To them, Beatrice—who was diminutive and spritely and whose countenance was open and accepting—was surely an enchanted being, living proof that fairy tales are real.

As in fairy tales, the theme of transformation was central to Beatrice's life. As a potter, of course, she was constantly transforming clay into objects of quiet but startling beauty. (There was never anything "extra" in a Beatrice pot; her pieces spoke to you, but never loudly; instead, they had the weight of real feeling, and they communicated that.) The transformation that she was more interested in, and that she devoted her life to, involved a much bigger and more profound work: the transformation of her being.

Beatrice began this work as a young woman in her 20s, when she met Solita Solano, another pupil of Gurdjieff's. Soon, she was living at Franklin Farms in New Jersey, a resident community of people who, like Beatrice, were searching to understand the meaning of their lives and how to live, authentically, a life based on values of a higher order.

In this search and in what it required—persistence, self-discipline, the constant wish to see and know oneself, an unflagging thirst for being—Beatrice was a natural. The influence of people she met at Franklin Farms—the de Hartmanns and Madame Ouspensky—never left her, even 60 years later. She was always applying her mind to the search. Beatrice wasn't a reader or, god forbid, a writer, but every day there was some intentional turning toward this question of how to live a more authentic life. She might copy out a quotation from a book and place it where it could serve as a frequent reminder, study one of the more challenging chapters in Gurdjieff's *All and Everything*, or step out into her garden and, with deep breaths, take it all in, intentionally. She was an avid swimmer well into her 80s, doing laps at the local pool, and also took up piano late in life.

Though Beatrice wasn't a writer, she did provide an account of her experiences with Gurdjieff during his last visit to America in 1949; it is published in her husband Frank's book *Without Benefit of Clergy*. To produce that account, she dictated while I typed, and it was an experience I will never forget. As Beatrice told her story, I would occasionally, without saying anything, make the smallest adjustment to a word or phrase in an effort to make it more grammatical or sound, to my mind, better (I did, after all, have some experience as an editor). But in reading a paragraph back to her, she knew in an instant when something had been changed. I would try to convince her, explain why it should be as I had written it, but she would have none of it. Just as she could, with that calm, steady, open gaze of hers, cut through lies, chatter, and masks, she could, by listening, hear a false note every time. Beatrice knew better than the editor how to keep the words authentic and real.

Perhaps this ability had something to do with having lived, for most of her life, so close to nature. Beatrice grew up on a dairy farm; there were the years at Franklin Farms; and then there was the house on the river in Grand View, where every spring Beatrice planted a vegetable garden. The idea was not to plant in rows separated by the proper amount of space, using the right amount of seed for each type of vegetable. No, when you planted with Beatrice, you learned that the point of having a vegetable garden was to extract as much nature as possible from the soil. So you doubled the number of rows and planted handfuls, rather than pinches, of seed. Everything grew, of course. It was riotous and unruly. That is, it was beautiful.

"The seed of God is in us," says Meister Eckhart, at the beginning of a quote that Beatrice loved. The quote was included in a little book of table graces that we often consulted before a meal together. In time, the Eckhart quote was the only one she wanted to hear, so I stopped trying to find others and would turn directly to it. Eventually, in keeping with that way she had of always applying herself, she and I enjoyed reciting it from memory. In the months after Beatrice died, I came to feel that the Eckhart quote—more than any biography that could be written about her—told the real story and significance of Beatrice's life, as well as what she taught me through being who she was. Said Meister Eckhart:

"The seed of God is in us. Given an intelligent and hard-working farmer, it will thrive and grow up to God, whose seed it is; and accordingly its fruits will be God-nature. Pear seeds grow into pear trees, nut seeds into nut trees, and God-seed into God."

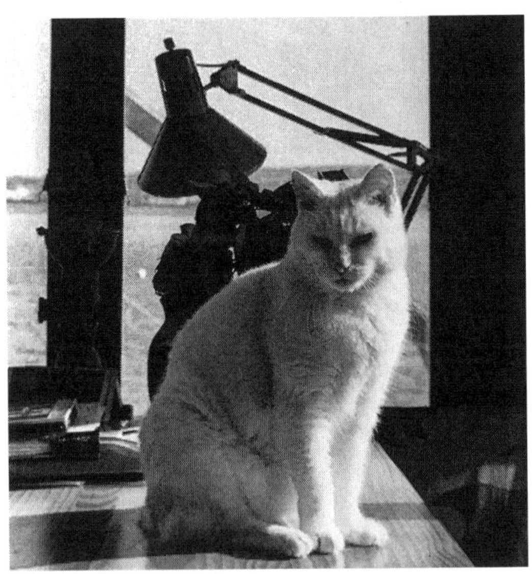

Beatrice's beloved house cat also found respite and beauty in the sun-filled porch on the Hudson.

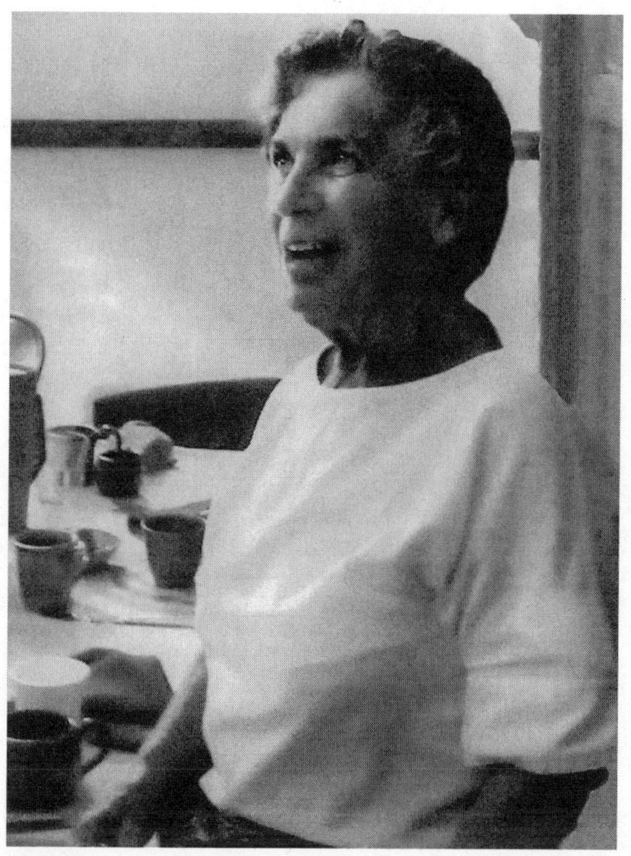

A prize-winning graduate of the Rhode Island School of Design, Beatrice was an artist who worked predominantly in clay.

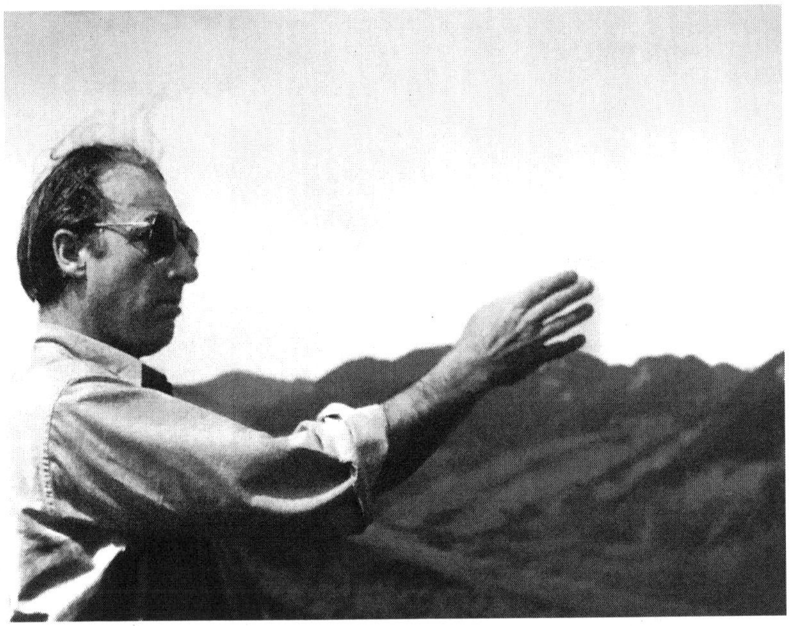

The author points out the trail to be negotiated on an early group hike in the Adirondacks.

# Part II:
# Reflections of the Real

# Introduction—First Section

I dare say that inserting two groups of so-called sittings—as I am doing in this book—is, as the saying goes, asking for trouble. It is an invitation to so much misunderstanding, misconception, presumption, betrayal, and blame.

I do not wish to reinforce the critics' arguments by sounding my own doubts and misgivings, but it should be understood that I am not trying to sound a kind of well-beloved longing for, or a hopeless declaration of, an unattainable reality.

Sittings encompassing a variety of methods and procedures have taken a central place in the Gurdjieff Work, beginning with Mr. Gurdjieff's teachers and Mr. Gurdjieff himself and followed for decades by Madame de Salzmann, who had initiated me into some of this subtle inner work. I won't try to describe a standard format or procedure. I see "sittings" as a rather deceptive term, since they are more like a preparatory positioning of the body, the mind and the feelings—indeed as "an opening toward the life aligned." Those who have worked with me in this manner will attest to the fact that I have pointedly—and unashamedly and often—declared that I have dutifully approached the sittings without, say, a prepared script. I have dutifully tried to work "in the moment," in the here and now. Indeed, I have acknowledged to those who work with me that my work in this format was unashamedly—to me—a "super effort."

In any event, for the purposes of this book I have arbitrarily divided these reports into two broad sections of sittings that took place over about six years at the New York Foundation. The first section dates back to January 2014 and ends in November 2018. The second, smaller section covers a shorter sequence of sittings, which had generally been held on Fridays with members of my own former groups and others. I recommend that, with both sections of sittings, the reader should ponder them one by one, and not altogether or in some rigid sequence. The truth is that the Work so revealed was truly part of an honest exploration shared by us all.

These transcripts have been rather randomly chosen. I recommend too that they be used individually. If they are used as a guide for an actual sitting, please be sure to maintain a certain tempo, and let the words and thoughts be heard.

# January 17, 2014—
# The Sense of Order

Perhaps we see more clearly now that our aim in working in this form, and in this way, is to become whole. It isn't to achieve some dramatic transformation on the spot, as it were. But to be whole I need to be centered. And I see that I cannot really begin this special inner effort without a certain sense of order. This order is needed because, as Mr. Gurdjieff reminds us, our parts are not related. And again, this order cannot be imposed or manipulated. It itself needs to be approached in an orderly and intelligent way.

Again Mr. Gurdjieff has given us an extraordinary indication of how to enter into this process. And his indication is that one needs to situate a center of gravity for the attention—in the abdomen. This is a kind of intentional intrusion into my, as it were, mechanicality, automaticity, whose extent and reach and hold I scarcely comprehend.

So I sense the need, again—which Mr. Gurdjieff brings to us in his special way—the need to occupy the body, the need to be, as it were, planted on the planet. And of course one's posture is critical. What kind of energies can I conceivably open to if I am all crooked and bent, slug-like? And I see that a growing sense of order begins to appear, because I allow it—I, as it were, step out of the way. One aspect of this sense of order is the sense of verticality. And the easing of the tensions in the thought, in the body. And through letting go of this attachment to *I* and *mine*, the opening now of the feeling. As I watch, as I witness this unfolding order, I can sense that these parts resonate at the same tempo, as one—and not in contention.

I begin to recognize that I belong to Presence, to this other current of life, quite distinct from the one through which I wish only to go out, to affirm, to affirm *me* and *mine*. I sense that I can't have both, and that this finer current is not accessible to that in me which thinks only of *me* and *mine*. And as this contact strengthens, because I am increasingly centered, I have the taste in moments of what it is to be void of the ego, this tyrant.

Again, I need to be intelligent—not to dream, not to think that I achieve. But I watch these movements, impartially. I witness the movement of energy, the movement of energies. I let them be... let them be. And who is this self, what is this self, that remembers? It is nothing that I create, it is uncreated. But I allow this opening, I allow this glimpse, this glimpse of the unknown.

I try not to put words to it. I watch, wordlessly, because there is a life beyond the constructs of the mind. To come to that in moments, to glimpse that, I need to trust the silence. And I quietly take stock: I'm aware of the sensation of the body, in the body, and I see that it is indeed a sign of obedience to what is finer. And I see too that perhaps for the first time, I can indeed say inside: *I Am*. And I can quietly follow the breath, as if I'm part of something greater that breathes. And I see too that what is so often and perhaps totally absent from my life is the sense of the transcendent and the real. I wish not to be shut from that. Again, for this I need to be liberated from the ego, which recognizes no master.

I see once again that to be whole requires that I be in touch with both these currents—this current of life that draws me out, and this current that descends, this conscious current that descends and reaches perhaps to the essence, if I allow it, if I stand out of the way.

But now we need to finish, so very intentionally I let this exploration cease, in order to go into life. And let us try to see if we can keep some thread of this work.

# December 12, 2014—
# The Need to Be Emptied

It has been said by the rare people who have come to this understanding that it is only when self—this self with a small "s," or what we know as the ego—it is only when this little self is eliminated from one's activities, or if you wish from one's thought, from one's feeling, from one's movements, that God can enter in. God, or consciousness. And surely if we are honest, and here we have to be honest—one has seen already in these opening minutes that we are indeed slaves of this ever-affirming ego, and this ever-affirming mind. The mind knows no master, and strangely it wants this continuity—through the thoughts, and the images, and the memories. And it is this incessant affirmation that prevents me from knowing who I am.

What we've understood—and Mr. Gurdjieff and Madame de Salzmann have made it so clear—that we cannot come to the unknown, to what is real, through the known. And it's because we are trapped in this way that we know only the illusion of who we are, of who I am. How then to enter yet again and again into this process by which I could open to what is real? I come to that not by forcing, by "doing," but rather through a process of opening and allowing this egoistic web to ease, to fall away.

So I need to be relaxed. At the same time a certain tension is needed. I relax in the thought, in the body, in the feeling. I open to the impression of being here now, being here now in this body. Very lightly, I'm aware of the breath, which is in itself an extraordinary exchange of energies. Without it, I would not exist. So I own to this fact, impartially, without thought or comment. And I see then I need to be in the present moment, now. And it is in the present moment that we human beings can act out our responsibility. And what is this responsibility? It is not merely to dream, to indulge, but to work for being. I wish to be more than just a verbal, mental, and emotional phantom.

I'm not doing anything, I'm simply watching, attending—wordlessly—to my present reality. This is not yet the real, but it is how I find myself. I let the thoughts flow, but I stay grounded in my atmosphere. I take in my whole situation with a kind of global overview. I am a witness in this present moment. At the same time as I work for this elusive quality of being, I do not pretend to be somebody or something. I wish to be open to the silence. It is the silence that encompasses all. And I have this inkling, this intimation, in moments, that I'm really opening to intelligence. But this intelligence is not here to serve me and my shallow ambition and my equally shallow understanding.

And slowly and almost imperceptibly and invisibly, a new order begins to take shape, a new relation between the head, the body, the feeling—again, not of my doing. In a sense I enable this by respecting the silence. And it is as if the head, the body, the feeling, resonate at the same tempo, and not at odds with each other—not in contention, not one dominating the other. And it is only now, then, that I can sense, as it were, a finer current, another current besides my temporal organic energy. And if you wish you may call this finer movement "presence." It is not my presence, but Presence.

One senses, then, one's role, the human being's role, which is to link these two currents—as it were, the horizontal and the vertical. And I see that I am, to my degree, in front of the unknown. I try to be there, here, without comment, without words, images, memories—void of thought, void of ego, empty. Again, because the unknown can't be known through the known. I see, then, that I am in front of a mystery, the mystery of who I am. And it is this direction in which I come to self-remembering. It's not me *and* my ego. As Madame reminds us, the Self, with a capital S, belongs to the Absolute. It is a very high thing, but I sense that I'm turned in this direction. I sense too that my real nature is consciousness. And of course I see the extent to which I betray that understanding and that trust. Once again I can come to what is real only by being emptied, emptied of myself.

As I said in the beginning, it's only through eliminating the me and the mine, the ego, that the higher, the real, can enter into one's actions. We don't see the enormity of the Work through our identification, which is relentless, unrelenting. So, then, to respect these moments of opening to what is real. And if we don't, who will? And as in the great traditions, Mr. Gurdjieff and Madame remind us, there is that in us (and it's not the ego), there is that in us which has this nostalgia to return to its primordial perfection. And this demands our uttermost—or, if you wish, a super effort. Not just lip service. It is a way, a real step, when I can accept to be unknowing—not to think, not to affirm the ego, but to respect that there is an intelligence at work in the universe.

And so, can I go into manifestation without totally losing this sense of the transcendent, which we see in looking around us is literally absent among our fellow men.

So let us finish.

# October 27, 2017—
# To Die to the Known

There are perhaps fifty ways of expressing what it is that we come together for. And so I will take one out of the hat, as it were, and see where this leads.

The one that I have in mind is one that Madame de Salzmann expressed so comprehensively when she said that we meet here and work here in order to die to the known. And what isn't understood terribly clearly is that we are by and large, and ordinarily, prisoners of our illusions—prisoners of the automatism, of the mechanical, of the automatic. So it is helpful, then, to enter into this exploration along the lines that Mr. Gurdjieff himself indicated.

I begin by detaching myself from what may be called the multiple, from all this stuff with which I am occupied and identified. It means that I need to find myself here, now, in this place, in this body, in this moment. Again, as Madame has put it so clearly, there is no time, only the present moment. And as Mr. Gurdjieff would put it, I begin by collecting my thoughts—his words: I collect my thoughts. Who am I? What am I? Where am I? And one sees that in order to undertake this exploration I need to enable a new order to appear between my so-called brains—the head, the body, the feeling. In a sense I locate them. Where is my thought? One sees that, by and large, it runs off. Then where is the body? And so I need, as it were, to establish its existence. I take in its verticality, its being grounded on the earth and offering a kind of conduit through me to what is beyond the head, because what we're trying to open to is a life beyond the constructs of the mind. And the third element in this, as it were, troika—the feeling. I *feel* the need to be.

And what we discover is that no one can do it for me—this inner work, this opening to what is real. And so I see I need to be still in all these parts—in the head, in the body, in the feeling. I can even undertake a very central exercise given by Mr. Gurdjieff right here in New York in 1948 on Christmas Day. What he urged those who were there was to connect to their breath, with their breathing. That when one breathes in, one quietly says "I"; and when I breathe out I quietly say "Am." Breath in "I," breathe out "Am." Not just once or twice, but I try to sustain this connection. And he added yet another wrinkle, as it were—and these are his words—that when I breathe in "I," it's as if something stands up inside. And when I breath out "Am," it's as if something sits down inside. And there is yet more that he indicated: that I allow each of these parts—the head, the body, the feeling—equal time, as it were. It's not one or the other, but all, equally.

And these are all extraordinary indications of the inner work for which we human beings have been created. It is said that we have been created in the image of God. And so our aim in our inner work is to become as God, to be deified. And this is an extraordinary demand. As Madame has put it, there is a cosmic need for the being that I wish to be. A cosmic need. It's not that I've been given this gift of life and this instrument simply to indulge myself. That is to miss the point; indeed it is criminal.

So I respect this inner silence and I respect the opening in me to the sense of *I Am*. And slowly one opens to the intimation that *I Am* is my real nature. I begin to listen to the resonance in me of *I Am*. It is nothing that I create. As I've mentioned here many times, *I Am* is at the very source of creation. As I've mentioned too, there is this marvelous story of Moses speaking to the burning bush. He had asked this burning bush, which had told him to return to the Israelites, "Who shall I say hath sent me?" And the voice in the burning bush said, "Say that *I Am* hath sent thee."

And over and above this, Mr. Gurdjieff indicated a very special exercise to establish the atmosphere around me. He indicated that this is an arm's length in each direction and that we need, as it were, to suck it in and sustain it. The point being that when this atmosphere is not intact, the atmosphere is dissipated.

So we are here to serve a very high purpose, a cosmic need. And this cannot be fulfilled so long as I am fragmented. It demands that I become whole. And already one knows that there is no sense of presence if I am not whole. So this is an extraordinary teaching. And I need to respect the silence. The silence is at the very source, and I need to stand unknowing before the unknown.

The Work is not a cheap thing. We are reminded again and again by Madame and Gurdjieff that the Self—this Self with a capital S—is a very high thing. It belongs, they have said, to the Absolute. I need to earn the right to open to that, to open to what is real. And what is real is void, empty, of the ego.

So we are called not only to separate ourselves from ourselves, but to empty ourselves of ourselves. This is no cheap thing. And so there are these moments in which one receives intimations of the timeless actuality of that which is transcendent. It is that which gives meaning to our lives. And I begin to listen to this resonance in me of *I Am*. Madame adds that in such moments the soul itself is here. And one begins to sense the need, as Gurdjieff reminds us, to pay for one's arising, to pay for this gift of life, and not simply to squander it in pointless affirmations of the ego.

So it's so important to have a work, not just here but in my day, and to try to remember when I go into manifestation that I am here to serve. So can we try then to keep this flame alive?

Very intentionally then, let us stop.

# November 3, 2017—
# The Taste of the Silence

I believe I am still correct in reminding us that when we come here and work together in this, as it were, format, we are not trying to "get" anything. And certainly we are not here to coddle our particular subjectivities in the name of Mr. Gurdjieff's Work. Rather, we need to die to what we have learned and what we know in order to open to what is unknown.

Perhaps that's as much as I might say, but I'll risk yet more. In a way, one might say that we aim to touch "a many-centered balanced-being perceptiveness," a need to which Mr. Gurdjieff himself has pointed us. And we can't really go too far afield if we enter into this exploration along the lines that Mr. Gurdjieff himself has indicated. He has pointed to the need for our so-called brains to be related, or if you wish, we need to be whole if we feel this need to open to what is real, to open to presence.

Mr. Gurdjieff himself has indicated to the groups he spoke to that one must collect one's thoughts. Those are his words—to collect one's thoughts. And that is a way of detaching oneself from thc multiple, and gathering one's energies here, in this moment. Because again, as we are reminded, there is no time, only the present moment, and the need is for each of us to find ourselves here, now. To respect the silence, to open to the silence. To locate, as it were, each of these brains. The head—where is it now? Its role is simply to register. The body—situating me on the planet, and through its verticality, opening to what is higher.

And the feeling—do I feel the need to have being?

Again, I respect the silence; I wish for the taste of the silence. I need to see that there is something in me, the ego, that is constantly affirming, affirming, and I say "I" to every affirmation. I need to stay in front of this mystery. As I've said, to die to what I know and what I have learned. And I allow these three brains their space. I see yet again this evidence that I am indeed a slave of the automatism, and I don't recognize it. I must accept yet another of the indications given by Mr. Gurdjieff: that I need a center of gravity for the attention. Otherwise it is taken at every turn by this automaticity, by my, as it were, machinery.

What I begin to acknowledge is this need to be emptied, this need to live in emptiness. I read recently that the Dalai Lama said that emptiness is consciousness. And what I begin to trust is that there is a life beyond the constructs of the mind. I must see how my energy, my attention, is taken, and I try not to go too far. I come back. And as I quieten, I begin to listen in me to the resonance of *I Am*. *I Am* is nothing that I create; it *is*.

And quietly I open to the extraordinary exchange of energies—the breathing. And quietly I can follow yet another indication given by Mr. Gurdjieff, which is that when I breathe in I say quietly "I," when I breathe out, quietly "Am." As I've reminded you, he even added a wrinkle—that when I say "I," it is as if something stands up in me. And when I say "Am," it is as if something sits down. Quietly I try to follow this, to be part of this extraordinary and invisible exchange. And as Madame would put it, it is as if the soul itself is present.

I continue to respect the silence. The silence is at the source. And the true silence is void of stuff, void of the ego, void of one's subjectivity. I try to stay related, continuing to watch the breath, not letting my thought wander off, not letting this voracious ego swallow everything. It swallows everything with its suffocating pretensions. And one begins to sense in moments that life, this extraordinary gift that each of us has received, is no cheap thing. We are here, as Mr. Gurdjieff tells us, to serve a very great purpose. And we have been created in the image of God. No less. And so one has these intimations in moments of this timeless actuality of that which is transcendent. And even in moments, one shares this understanding that "life is real only then, when *I Am*."

And so one has the taste in moments of what it means to die to the known in order to enter the unknown. And how to carry that recognition into manifestation? As I remind us all, as Madame has reminded us in turn, there is a cosmic need for the being that I would wish to be, for the being that each of us would wish to be. This is nothing to do with one's subjectivity, with *me*.

And so now, very intentionally, I leave this and go into manifestation, wishing to continue to serve honorably and unselfishly. So let us finish.

# December 8, 2017—
# To Live in Emptiness

There are probably fifty different ways of entering into this exploration in which we are joined. It's good to see so many of you have come. And I will therefore venture to say that what we are entering into is no idle pursuit. As Madame de Salzmann has put it so beautifully, there is a cosmic need for the being that I would wish to be. A cosmic need. Not some little stunt to gloss over my subjectivities and weaknesses and ambitions and illusions.

Because again we need to be reminded that we are ordinarily slaves of the automatism. And our overriding aim is really to die—again as Madame puts it—to die to the known in order to open and enter into the unknown. How then to enter into this extraordinary work, a work for which Mr. Gurdjieff himself has said that we need to have "all-brained balanced-being perceptiveness"?

Mr. Gurdjieff was extraordinarily, shall I say, prescient in indicating how one should enter into such an undertaking. And he gave some very, very precise indications. To begin with, I, as it were, detach myself from the multiple, the fragmentation in myself. And to use Gurdjieff's words, "I collect my thoughts"—to establish that I am here, now, in this place, in this moment, in this body. I need to be very, very still in all the parts—in the head, the body, the feeling. And the point is that I cannot come to what is real, I cannot open to what is real, until these parts come into a new order, a new relation. Presence is inaccessible to the thought by itself, or the feeling by itself.

So already I am occupied in a new way. I must respect the silence. I do not allow my thoughts to wander. I can follow the breath, which in itself is an extraordinary exchange of energy. And slowly and quietly and wordlessly I listen to the resonance in me of *I Am*. Madame de Salzmann says that "it is the soul itself" that is here when I can open and listen to that special resonance. The *I Am* is nothing that I create; it *is*.

I can also then echo another of Mr. Gurdjieff's special and extraordinary indications of how to work in this all-brained balanced-being way of perceiving. Mr. Gurdjieff gave that indication here, at Christmas, 1948. That when I breathe in I quietly say "I," when I breathe out I quietly say "Am." And he added yet another aspect, which was that when I breathe in, it is as if something stands up. When I breathe out, it is as if something sits down. And you see when you follow indications like that, that one is indeed dying to the known and opening to the unknown.

And so I guard this inner silence. I try not to be taken too far by a thought, by an image, by some memory, by some tension in me. I need to be totally relaxed.

I guard the energy. When I am still I can follow the movement of the energies in me, and meet them before they take a form. So what we are encountering now in this way is, as it were, evidence that we have been created as human beings to serve a very great purpose. I am not here on the planet, in this body, simply to indulge my appetites, or my wish to be important, the top dog. Because I am here to serve. And it is said in all of the great traditions—and Mr. Gurdjieff is no exception—that we have been created "in the image of God." And so life, this life that we are encountering, is an extraordinary gift.

Almost imperceptibly, then, I open to the actuality of that

which is real, of that which is transcendent. And it can be known only through dying to the known, dying to my dream, dying to the illusion that I am somebody. And so I have the inkling now that I am here in this body, on the planet, to become as God. Gurdjieff, in his Christmas Day exercise, said, "Become Christ." So our work is really to be deified, to become as God, to become whole. So I respect this impression of being whole. And for that, I need to be emptied, emptied of *me* and *mine*. I must learn to live in emptiness.

And I have these intimations now again, as Madame de Salzmann put it so clearly, that there is no time, only the present moment. And I see the need to be in the present moment. I need to find myself again and again, here, now, in this place, in this body. To stand unshakably in the true. What an extraordinary gift.

I continue to listen to the resonance in me of *I Am*. Again, I don't invent or create *I Am*. It *is* before I was. Even now, I check my posture and I value the sense of verticality that indicates that I am indeed a conduit of unknown energies, very high energies. And through these efforts I pay for my arising, I pay for the extraordinary gift of being born a human being.

So I have again renewed my commitment to serve that which is Real.

And without abandoning this fragile connection to what is transcendent, I try to sustain this connection as I go into manifestation.

Let us very intentionally end this effort and go into life as we know it. Let us stop.

# April 20, 2018—
# The Need to Become Whole

When we come together like this, it is not to get anything or achieve anything, or to reinforce our subjectivities. Rather, it is to open to the real. And of course each time we come together is a new moment. How then to enter into this extraordinary exploration? I take Madame de Salzmann at her word when she says that when we come here, our overriding aim is to die to the known.

You can find your own "knowns," and make your own definitions, but our aim is to die to all of the assumptions and dreams and illusions that we reinforce through the way that we live. To die indeed to the known. And then the truth is that everything in which we are immersed and engaged is unknown. And as I've said often when we come together, Mr. Gurdjieff gave very, very clear indications of how to enter into this exploration—very clear, very precise. So what we are called to face is the need to become whole. Because as we are, we are fragmented, divided.

And if the aim of a teaching such as Mr. Gurdjieff's and the great revelations is to bring about normality, we have to enter into this exploration in a completely different way from the way we ordinarily live. Because the truth is—as these great teachers have pointed out—that God created man in order that man could become God. This is a very high aim. It has nothing to do with enhancing one's ego, one's position. Nothing to do with indulging one's subjectivities, one's weaknesses, ambitions.

So we begin by accepting to be in question: Who am I? What am I? And Mr. Gurdjieff was very clear that one must begin, as he put it, by collecting one's thoughts, to ascertain that I am indeed here, now, in this place, in this body, in this moment. As Madame reminds us, there is no time, only the present moment.

And may I point out that this demands that you guard your postures—you're leaning over backwards, sideways. What kind of energy results from that? And this opens one to ideas that are very central to this teaching. As the thought quietens, as I detach myself from what has been called the multiple—all these fragments that course through me and with which I identify—I begin to open, and to listen, to the resonance in me of *I Am*. It is here; nothing that I create, but something that I can open to. And slowly there is this sense that the *I Am* resonates in all my parts, undivided.

And it is only through this, as it were, cohesive resonance in me that I'm able to open in moments to a sense of presence. I can't, as it were, bring it about simply by thinking, or by feeling, or through the tensions in the body. And then I begin to sense that *I Am*, I have been created as a three-brained human being, in the image of God. So that life is not just a cheap thing—I am here to serve, to serve a very great and unknown purpose. As Madame, again, has put it, there is a cosmic need for the being that I would wish to be. And then again, to keep us honest, we need to recognize and acknowledge that as we ordinarily live, we are slaves of the automatism. The automatism affirms itself at every turn. And I say "I" to each of these manifestations, each of these affirmations. So I need to trust the silence, I need to accept that I am unknowing, in order to enter into the unknown. I must do this wordlessly, without these endless churnings of one's subjectivity, of one's wish to be recognized.

And I need to learn how to serve this unknown reality that lies beyond the constructs of the mind.

And so I listen. I wish to differentiate between the real—this timeless actuality of what is transcendent—and on the other hand, all the stuff that goes on in my mind. Because the truth is I am being called. And the silence is at the source. I need to respect its existence, its presence, its reality.

I try to keep the space. I don't need the images and memories, because it is an extraordinary thing to find myself here in this moment. It opens me to the sense of what prayer is—to stand, as it were, in the presence of God. And that is really what we are being called to learn: how to pray. Indeed, as these marvelous monks of old, and of our times, try—to pray without ceasing. For that I need to be emptied, emptied of *me* and *mine*. And it begins, as Mr. Gurdjieff pointed out, by separating myself from myself. He points out that that is something an adult can do. And I continue that, deepen that, by emptying myself of myself. And I have the taste in moments that the self does indeed belong to the Absolute. It is a very high thing. And I've been created to enable that. So I have an inkling in moments of what it must mean to die to the known.

And I devote myself to discerning and differentiating between that which is real and that which is not. So this is a very high calling, a very high service. And I see the need, which Mr. Gurdjieff exemplified, the need to occupy this body, to inhabit it, to carry the sense of this verticality—that I am indeed a conduit for energies that flow to and from a very high source.

And so, as we leave this in a minute or two, can we try to be in touch with this unknown world that lies beyond the constructs of the mind? I respect it through my silence, through my acceptance of the unknown. And as I can, I try to listen to the resonance in me of I *Am*. It *is*, it is here, it's not an invention.

It's an extraordinary reality that I know only in moments.

So we've been given a very great gift in having this extraordinary being to occupy. Can we keep something of that alive as we go into manifestation?

And so now, very intentionally, I go into movement.

# June 1, 2018—
# Opening to the Life Force

There must be an infinite number of points of entry into the exploration that we are attempting in coming together in this way. But the one that has struck me ever more in recent times is Madame de Salzmann's indication that we should "die to the known."

It is hard to imagine anything as encompassing as that. To die to the known. And the truth is, I believe, that we can't come to that knowledge unless, and until, we are whole. And so together we need to search inwardly for the way to work for that. Of course the way needs to be encountered, discovered, explored, here, now. It is outside of time. And as Madame reminds us, there is no time, there is only the present moment. And how then to enter into that?

As I've reminded us Friday regulars, as it were, Mr. Gurdjieff was very clear about how to begin. Reading his lectures and recollections of his talks and exchanges, one sees that he gave very, very precise indications of how to enter into this exploration. How, in fact, to die to the known. And the truth is, the known is actually a mystery, actually unknown. So he made it clear that I need, we need, to collect ourselves. He actually said to "collect one's thoughts." After all, why am I on the planet, what am I, who am I? This is something that I encounter for myself, now. I see that I have to be still, I need to trust the silence, to accept not knowing.

And as I've mentioned, one of the great Platonic minds of our time [Frithjof Schuon] has given an extraordinary indication—that I begin by detaching myself from the multiple, from all these thoughts and ideas and memories and attachments. I try to let them be, let them go. I try not only to separate myself from myself, but I also try quietly, intelligently, to empty myself of myself—all these old memories and attachments and illusions.

And I see what is needed—it's not my invention. This comes from our great teachers, that I want my three brains, as it were—the head, the body, the feeling—to be aligned and not in competition. After all, it should be no surprise to be reminded, in fact, that, as I am, I am a slave of the automatism. It affirms itself unceasingly and unconsciously, and without knowing it, I say "I" to every affirmation. So I open, I detach myself from this insistent, endless, and unintelligent affirmation. Because I have this inkling now, through such efforts, that my real nature is consciousness.

I try to stay, as it were, in front of this recognition. If I'm taken by a memory, an image, a thought, a tension, I try not to go too far. And almost imperceptibly, I listen to the resonance in me of another life. I don't give it a name—I don't compare, I try to stay, unmoving, and empty. I'm not working for some result. And I see that I'm opening to something extraordinary, that it is the *I Am* that resonates in my parts. It is nothing that I create. It is. It is before I was. And I accept to be unknowing. I accept to be, as it were, dying to what I believe I know, in order to enter the unknown.

And as I've indicated many times, what this kind of effort opens one to is the centrality of *I Am* in Mr. Gurdjieff's work. And it is that that I wish to open to and to serve. What an extraordinary mystery. Because what one is receiving an inkling of is an opening to what is real, an opening to the life force.

And I see how I block that with my stupid identifications, my unintelligent so-called inner world.

But what we're invited to do is to open instead to a new and unknown intelligence. And that comes through the feeling. It can't be felt if I am identified, if I'm simply dreaming. So I watch my posture and to be erect, pure. We're engaged in a process of purification, a process of opening to what is real.

I am reminded that I was in the house in Mendham the night that Madame Ouspensky died, and three days later we received an extraordinary letter from Madame de Salzmann. And part of it is in her book. I don't know how the editor came to stick it right in the middle of some alien passage, but in it Madame said, "There is no death, life cannot die." And it is to this that we are orienting ourselves in working as we do, to be conscious occupants of this human entity. And as we become more and more sensitive, we have the taste at times of that which both Madame de Salzmann and other teachings describe as *nostalgia*, nostalgia for the primordial origins of who we are. We are in fact, as it were, sparks of God. It has been said that God created man in order that man could become God. Which is no cheap thing. It's an extraordinary gift, this gift of life.

And so when I listen to the resonance in myself of *I Am*, it is the soul with which I am linked. You find Madame speaks, writes, in her book, about that. The soul is here. How then to sustain this intensity? So it's so important that we have a work. And especially a work to have a center of gravity, a center of gravity for the attention, which is of course an aspect of consciousness.

So forgive me for launching us afield, but if we don't work in this way, who will? If we don't aspire to be as God, who will? And you may remember that when Mr. Gurdjieff gave that marvelous exercise with the *I Am* back in 1948 here in New York, he urged people to "Become Christ." He said, "Be." So we have this extraordinary work to grow the being, and there is clearly a cosmic need for this activity, a *cosmic* need.

Can we then, without throwing everything to the wind, can we keep the sense of this order, keep the sense of it when I go into manifestation? It would be a way of paying for one's arising. So let us very intentionally finish this and go out into life, carrying this understanding. It's an extraordinary gift, and we wish to learn how to pay for it.

So let us stop.

# November 9, 2018—
# The Need for Inner Order

With so many, as it were, points of entry, it is always a question of where to begin. My own inclination is to approach an occasion like this in Madame de Salzmann's extraordinary terms—that we are here to die to the known. She also makes it clear—and I would like to quote her exact words—"When I work in the quiet, I do not let myself begin without an order being established around my center of gravity."

And then there are almost endless reasons for entering into a search like that. Because I'm not here to achieve, or to get, or to escape. I'm here to work for being. And what we discover—some of us, perhaps never—is that we are slaves of this automatism which endlessly and persistently affirms itself. And to each affirmation we say "I," "I." We do not see that we are slaves of a voracious egotism. And so Mr. Gurdjieff and Madame and a few other souls emphasize that we work in such a way that we can be unburdened of the ego. How indeed to come to that?

So once again one discovers that the obstacle to this freedom, to this growth of being that we wish, is right at hand. What is needed is really to have a center of gravity. And Mr. Gurdjieff clearly favored situating this center of gravity in the lower abdomen. It is there, he said, that the first body, this body, is connected to the second, to the astral. And this is yet elusive unless I pay attention to my posture, and ensure that I'm erect. And to a certain extent, but not only, to be relaxed.

Because I need to see where I am, I need to ask, Who am I? I've been given this extraordinary gift of life, and an extraordinary instrument to house it.

It is said that we are created in the image of God. And so I need to verify what I can, which is that I do have three brains: the head, the body, the feeling. And this is nothing that I take for granted. I need, as it were, to establish their existence. The head here, the body here, on the earth, and acting as a channel, a vertical axis, to energies that are above us, above the head. Those energies are deposited there through the efforts, the conscious efforts, of those who work intelligently.

And then thirdly, the feeling. It is the feeling that opens me to the intelligence that indicates a special work to be conscious. And even now I need to watch my posture, verify my so-called presence. And even now, in moments, I can listen to the resonance in me of *I Am*. And the *I Am* is very central to this teaching. It is nothing that I create. Rather, I open to its timeless actuality.

All of this needs to be verified, checked, corroborated, without words, innerly. So I have this inkling then that I am opening to a real world beyond the constructs of the mind. And so Madame's indication that one needs to die to the known is an extraordinarily encompassing vision. And it can only be, as it were, undertaken, corroborated, in the present. As Madame points out so well, there is no time, there is only the present moment. And I need to find myself here, now. Not at some future time, but now. And I try not to write any [inner] documents at this moment. I wish to be still. I wish to be unknowing. I wish not to intrude. I wish to have being. And then one sees that it is only when I die to all I know that I can open to something new. I'm not here to seek, or achieve gratification, or pleasure, or an escape.

And one can quietly follow the breath. As I've reminded you,

Mr. Gurdjieff brought this particular exercise to New York, at Christmas 1948. He indicated that one could, at the moment, breathe in and say "I," and breathe out and say "Am." He even said that when I breathe in "I," it's as if something stands up inside. When I breathe out "Am," it's as if something sits down inside. I quietly follow the breath, breathing in "I," breathing out "Am," quietly. And there come these extraordinary moments in which I allow what is transcendent in me to act. It is the *I Am* that is transcendent. And it acts through each of these parts. And there come these moments when all the parts—head, body, feeling—resonate at the same tempo, as the *I Am*. I try not to manipulate, or fake, but I try to be whole. I try to be three-brained. And it is only then that I truly open to what is real, as if I am learning to pray. And it is a big opening to be able to stand, as it were, in the presence of God. So this is such an extraordinary work, this work to be conscious and to come to conscience. And we must own to the fact that we truly betray what is sacred in the way we ordinarily live. I am here to serve a very high purpose.

And so it is not totally irrelevant to be reminded that Mr. Gurdjieff emphasized this central need to open to what is real. And as he would say, Life is real only then, when *I Am*. I'm trying to emphasize that the *I Am* is something beyond the ego. Real I is void of the ego. So how then to be faithful to this obligation that we have to work for being? Not for my gratification or pleasure, but in order that I pay for my arising. And the truth is, as Madame reminds us, that when I am situated in my center of gravity there is no ego that imprisons me.

So when we go out into manifestation try to have some sense that life is real only then, when *I Am*. And to allow this transcendent reality to act in me, through me. And to have some connection; not to squander it all, but to come back again and again. To accept to be unknowing. Because it's only in that way that one can enter into the unknown.

So let us stop, but try to keep some thread.

# Introduction—
# Second Section

The following transcripts are of sittings I conducted before an audience of no more than thirty-five people generally on Fridays with members of my own groups and others. They should be read (or used) in the order in which they occurred, because the perceptive reader will sense a certain progression or development. Indeed, I subtly inserted a certain progressive unfolding that will be evident from the insertion of "new" terms such as *individuation*—a particular unfolding favored by Carl Jung—and references to "advanced" terminology such as the *mundus imaginalis*, the extraordinary contribution of Henry Corbin.

Note: I had intended a unique insertion for the previous section's November 9, 2018 reflection. The insertion was a sitting which I had been asked to conduct at the Gurdjieff Foundation of New York's Lake work center several years prior and that left a deep impression of the need to open to the unknown. Paul Reynard, who was co-president of the Foundation with me at the time, was present and seated on a cushion on the floor to my right. I recall that as I approached the room, I was quietly informed that news had been received that Paul's son had died in an airplane crash in Brazil the night before. Rather than disturb the proceedings by introducing this information, and given that Paul chose to remain in silence where he sat, I subtly adjusted my presentation so as to include this newest unknown in the whole. When the sitting ended about forty minutes later, we all left the room without a further word being said. It was only then that I had a chance to speak to Paul and to quietly offer my condolences. My sitting appeared to have embraced the situation and to have helped us all to open—wordlessly—to the great Unknown.

# December 14, 2018—
# A Subtle Intelligence

Please understand that I do not have a script. I say that again because one takes one's lead from someone like Madame de Salzmann, who reminds us that we are here to die to the known. And it is something that we cannot profess to command. At the same time, we are not here to get anything or to achieve anything. Rather—let me put it rather bluntly—we are here to understand the nature of silence. And that is not a cheap thing.

As I also remind us, when we come together like this, there is a reality beyond the constructs of the mind. And that reality does not exist simply to serve the ego. It is good to be reminded, and to verify—as I can—that one is indeed a slave of the automatism. It is this automatism, this automaton, which endlessly affirms itself. And I, in my ignorance and lack of will, say "I" to every affirmation.

We've been around for some time, so that we know that these affirmations are, as it were, expressions of the thought, of tensions in the body, and a very low-level order of feeling. I like, I don't like. So how to give what is needed to this study? A study that would open this understanding—that silence enables—I can begin right here: I check my posture, I need to be erect, still. And Mr. Gurdjieff and Madame remind us that when we enter into this work that we are attempting now, a certain order needs to appear between my parts. I verify, as it were, that I have a thinking center, a moving center, and a feeling center. And I try to be still, erect—outwardly, inwardly. I try not to be taken by a tension, a reaction, a thought. Can I try indeed to be empty? The Dalai Lama tells us that emptiness is consciousness. And I need to try to open to this understanding. Almost imperceptibly I sense the movement in myself of *I Am*. It is nothing that I create. It is. It is at the very source. And I see that I am indeed in front of the unknown.

I try not to inject, insert, impose anything. But watch your postures, please. These extraordinary and subtle and deep energies need a certain purity of the posture—relaxed, but yet with the right tension. And again, almost imperceptibly, I sense—in fact, I *feel*—the presence of a very subtle intelligence which needs the space, which needs the stillness, which needs the attention. So I'm not doing, but rather *opening* as I can to a reality beyond the constructs of the mind. And this is not a cheap thing. It's nothing that I can achieve through our usual "group-think." It is something that only each of us individually can open to. And at the same time, each of us is supported by the real efforts of those around us.

As I've said, this is not a cheap thing, and it is an extraordinary gift to have been given this human form. I need to wake to its existence, its presence. And we've been created, it is said in the great revelations, we have been created in the image of God. Clearly then, we are here to serve a very great purpose—something one wishes to understand wordlessly, in silence, here in this moment, in this body. And slowly then, I receive an inkling of this extraordinary reality as I listen to the resonance in me of *I Am*. And I sense then that these parts resonate as one, together, as a whole.

Try not to talk to yourself, try not to chase some image, some memory, but accept to be here, in this present moment. Madame reminds us that there is a cosmic need for the being that I would wish to be. A cosmic need—nothing to do with my petty egoism, my subjectivity. And that which is real is not here to serve or to enhance my egoism. And I accept to be unknowing. I'm not here to invent and to impose, but rather, I accept to be unknowing in order to enter the unknown.

So one sees that this is indeed an extraordinary teaching. And we should not settle in ourselves for some cheap gratification of the ego. The real I is void of the ego. And here we are, created in the image of God—in order to become as God. Or as the scholars say, this work is for deification. It's not here for my cheap gratification. And there's all this cheap talk about the "conscious ego." So I see I need a center of gravity for the attention. Otherwise I'm simply a slave of the automaton, the equipage.

So I try to keep the sense, the sense that I need to serve a very great purpose. I'm here to pay for my arising. And I must respect the silence which is at the very source. And so, when we finish this exercise, can we move with some discernable respect for that which is transcendent in us, respect for that which is, for that which is *felt* as *I Am*? It helps to remember Mr. Gurdjieff's extraordinary gift in pointing out that "Life is real only then, when 'I Am.'"

So let us finish, and let us remember.

# January 18, 2019—
# Work to Be Whole

I suppose that each of us is accepting of the fact that, like Ashiata Shiemash, we need to work for all-centered balanced-being perceptiveness. Or as Mr. Gurdjieff emphasized, we need to become whole. We need also to acknowledge that we are actually slaves of the automaton, which endlessly affirms itself automatically. And we in our ignorance and our lack of understanding and lack of will say "I" to each of these affirmations. Which is why we need to begin to recognize and acknowledge the need not only for silence but also the need to acknowledge what is real.

And the need to be emptied is very much related to something that the Dalai Lama has said. And what he said was that "emptiness is consciousness." And so there's no shame in being empty, especially of the idiocy and lunacy and presumptiveness that one nurtures. So we come then to this extraordinary thought that Madame de Salzmann emphasized, that we need to die to the known in order that we may enter into the unknown. And that is something I can engage in, right now—not to be talking and arguing and proving inside, but to accept to be still, to be still in all the parts, all the brains, as it were: the head, the body, the feeling. And that need to be still opens me to what is real, to that which is. It enables that in me which is related to the source—it enables *that* to act.

And the truth is that what acts is the *I Am*. In moments, I can listen to the resonance in me of *I Am* in the parts—in the head, in the body, in the feeling. As Madame points out, it's through the resonance that I can actually tell that the soul is here—which is a very deep thing. But I need to be still, unknowing. And the thought, especially, needs to be still because the truth is that there is a real life beyond the constructs of the mind and these thoughts.

And so I need to be attentive to my posture, ensuring that it be aligned, vertical. Because I am a kind of conduit to that which is finer and higher. And the truth is that in moments one can actually, as it were, access this finer energy, which is lodged above us, through our efforts and the efforts of others. I need to trust and open to this silence, because it is true that our thinking cannot commune with the unknown. So this is an extraordinary possibility, that we can die to the known. But not by pushing it away, but rather by opening to the unknown.

So I wish to be open to the energy which courses through me. Just the energy, not my interpretations or my inner propaganda about my status or lack of same. And this is an extraordinary gift, this gift of life that I've received. And truthfully, I have a responsibility to guard that precious—I would say, that precious "stuff." But I don't guard it through talking, through proving, through trying to achieve or get. And so truthfully I'm here, as is each of us, to serve a very great and ultimately unknown service. And yes, another of these astonishing thoughts: that there is a cosmic need—*a cosmic need*—for the being that I would wish to be. It's not about getting something for myself, for me, but to serve a very high purpose in the scheme of things.

And so I come in moments to this inkling that there is a timeless actuality of the transcendent in me. A timeless actuality. Because again we are reminded by these extraordinary people—Madame, Mr. Gurdjieff—that there is no time, only the present moment. And this is where I need to situate myself: here, now, in this body, in this moment. And I see then, I have glimpses then, that I'm involved, as it were, in a process of deification, or if you wish, of becoming like God. This is a mark of all of the great revelations, this special role that is assigned. And again, I have this sense of the resonance in myself, in my parts, of the *I Am*. It is nothing that I create. It IS, it IS before I was. And I see I have this privilege of enabling it to act in me and in my parts. And I have the inkling of what it is to be whole.

It's an extraordinary teaching and it is an extraordinary privilege to be together as we are, to enter as and if we can, into the unknown.

And so we see that we must die to the known. I must die to my so-called known in order for this priceless unknown to be revealed. And so I see that I need not merely capitulate to what Madame calls my, our, ferocious—I repeat: ferocious—egotism.

So it is so good and so right that we come together as we do, to work to be whole. And it is only through being whole that I can open to presence and to what is real. So can we try simply to take in this actuality, this timeless actuality of that which is real, without trying to do or manipulate, and acknowledge this need to serve, to pay for this extraordinary gift of life.

And when I end and I go into manifestation can I carry something of this invisible actuality with me, acknowledging this extraordinary privilege of being given life, and not to be misled by the illusoriness of, as it were, planetary life. And so I try to carry with me this sense that I am activated by *I Am*, remembering Moses and the burning bush, when he said to the bush: "Who shall I say hath sent me?" The voice said, "Say that *I Am* hath sent thee." Perhaps I could truly be a servant of the Lord. And so let us finish.

# February 22, 2019—Silence at the Source

When we come together like this, it isn't to get anything, it isn't to achieve anything. And it is not to do anything in the way that we ordinarily face our lives. Just to clear the decks, I must admit to you that I do not have a prepared text—but we have so many of Mr. Gurdjieff's very, very precise indications of what is expected of us when we come together on an occasion like this.

For example, he has indicated the need for all-brained balanced-being perceptiveness in an encounter such as we are hoping to undertake here, now, together. Which is in itself an extraordinary indication of what is lacking, and of what is needed, when we undertake perhaps the most central effort that he puts before us—which is to make certain efforts, if you wish, to be whole.

And this is really the primary confirmation that we are called to affirm that we've been given our extraordinary gift of life and the extraordinary gift of, as it were, multiple brain systems. And we begin to sense that this is no idle gift—it's an extraordinary gift, to enable the parts to come into a real relationship. One takes one's lead from what Gurdjieff and Madame de Salzmann have given us: that there is no time, only the present moment.

Again, in going through Mr. Gurdjieff's material, one sees how very, very precise he is in indicating how one needs to begin. So I'm not here to get or to achieve or to enhance my, as it were, external positioning. I'm here to enable a real growth of being.

So I put aside my customary infatuation with my subjectivity. As I've told you many times, I'm guided by a discovery made decades ago. I described this to Madame de Salzmann and she said to me, "That is Real I." And I can assure you that a very central feature of that state of being is that it is void of the ego, void even of ethnicity. So how to approach, how to meet this moment in a new way? Not as a slave of my customary egoism, not as a slave of my mechanicality, not as a slave of my voracious egoism, of which we are reminded again and again and again. Because what we are called to investigate, to explore, in coming here like this is the actuality of the real, the actuality of that which is transcendent.

And so my undertaking is to open to what is Real. This is a very exacting exploration. I don't sit here and argue with myself and write long inner dissertations. But rather, I open to the silence. It is the silence that is at the source. And we can have tastes in moments of this actuality, because it's so central to Mr. Gurdjieff's teaching—this overriding actuality of *I Am*. It is nothing that I invent, nothing that I argue about. But in moments I taste it. In fact, in moments as I grow quieter and as I become more whole, I open to the resonance in me of *I Am*. Again, this is nothing that I invent or that I apply almost posthumously. Because the *I Am* is at the very heart of this extraordinary teaching. When I simply try to be still in the body, in the head, in the feeling, I actually enable the *I Am* to act.

Just to give us a little orientation, Mr. Gurdjieff and others have told the story of Moses and the burning bush. Moses asked the voice in the burning bush, on being told that he should go back to the Israelites, "Who shall I say hath sent me?" And the voice in the burning bush said, "Say that *I Am* hath sent thee." So one takes this seriously. I put my reactive thoughts aside, and my bellyaches and my reactions, and I open to what is Real. And

I take seriously what Mr. Gurdjieff has indicated to us, that we are ordinarily slaves of the automatism. It is the automatism that is ceaselessly affirming itself. And to each affirmation I blindly say I, I, I.

I can quote Madame again when she says that everything that reinforces the ego brings division, isolation. And at the same time I must watch my body. I want to be erect. Just the slightest departure from a certain purity in my posture spoils this inner vision. And again, Madame has said that everything I wish needs to be paid for. If I wish to have a new state I must sacrifice the old. So again, as Madame has put it to us, there is a cosmic need for the being I would wish to be. A cosmic need. It is nothing of my invention, or yours. We are here to serve. And we are here to find out how to serve. It is no cheap thing. And so what we begin to confirm in the way we work and value the silence is that there is a life beyond these little constructs of my mind. A real life.

And in one of her truly insightful remarks, Madame reminds us of something in all of the great revelations: that we have a nostalgia for that life. It is not a cheap thing that we are being called by it. And so I see that there is this real being obligation to serve. I open to that by dying to the known. This is an extraordinary call. And I can meet it only consciously. So I need the attention, I respect the attention. And as Gurdjieff points out, we need a center of gravity for the attention. Otherwise it is taken by every reaction, every dream, every identification.

So as I said earlier, as I reminded us in the toast on the thirteenth of January, there is a real need then to die to the known. It is something that I undertake in the present—not next week, next year, but now. And I stand unknowing before that. I'm not here to substitute a new interpretation, which is just another activity of my thought, of my automatism. I must die to the known in order to enter the unknown. This is such extraordinary material. And as I've reminded you, the Dalai Lama has said that emptiness is consciousness. How then to live in emptiness?

Some of you may remember that that was the title of a book that was printed at Armonk: *To Live in Emptiness*. And I accept to be unknowing, as opposed to inserting all of my stuff, inflicting my stuff. How then to sustain this differentiation between the real and the unreal? I must see that this lies in the extraordinary necessity to be emptied of one's egoism. Not to indulge this ferocious mechanicality. And I try to carry this with me, this need, because at the heart of it is the work that all the great revelations point to, which is the work for deification, to become as God. What an extraordinary exploration and what an extraordinary service.

And so, as we leave this quiet work and go into manifestation, try to keep some, as it were, contact with this unknown world of *I Am*. And thank you for coming. But to keep some thread of the effort.

# March 8, 2019—
# Not to Be a Slave

I must confess that I have no formal prepared script to guide us, as it were, into the unknown. But I'm glad to know that we've entered into this extraordinary exploration together many times.

And one begins to trust the overriding thrust of what we undertake in coming together in this form, on these occasions. And of course, at the risk of great repetition, I can think at this moment of nothing more compelling than to take up Madame de Salzmann's extraordinary indication that the thrust of what we attempt here now is to die to the known. This is not an undertaking that someone else will do on my behalf—but it is an investigation, an exploration, that only I can undertake for myself. And we can't do better than to accept the guidance that Mr. Gurdjieff has provided: that the work here is that I try to become whole.

I've been given this extraordinary gift of life, and it is said in the great revelations that we have been created in the image of God. Of course, what we discover when we begin this inquiry is that we are not whole, that the parts—these extraordinary brains—are not related. And so I must begin. And once again Madame is so clear in what she conveys, that there is no time, only the present moment. How then to locate myself as a three-brained entity wishing to fulfill a cosmic need? A cosmic need—not my pathetic, egoistic ambition.

And this work to die to the known situates that voracious entity, the egoism, right at the center of this undertaking. We've come to realize, in our sane moments, that we are ordinarily simply slaves of this automaticity, slaves of this egoism. And I want not to be a slave. I wish on the contrary to serve. And what we've begun to suspect and corroborate is precisely that—that we are here not to be slaves, but to be in the service of a very great purpose largely unknown to us.

So one needs to establish that one is here in this place, in this body, in this moment, respecting the source, the silence, the emptiness. So it's very important how I am situated physically. And one begins to see the—as it were—means of communication within one. And this bodily sensation is not the least of those means. It's perhaps at the very center, because I wish to be free of these tensions, in all the parts. I wish to respect the silence, respect not knowing, respect this extraordinary indication that I am here to grow in being.

This is not a cheap thing, it really has nothing to do with the seeming glamor of my subjectivity. So I need to come to a fundamental tranquility, to be without these tensions, without avidity, greed, acquisitiveness. And slowly I begin to listen to the resonance in me of that which animates us all. Gurdjieff speaks a great deal about the role and the place of *I Am*. It is nothing that I invent, *it Is*. And as I begin to differentiate in myself between the imaginary and the real, I begin to listen to the resonance in me of the *I Am* as it acts in me. When these parts resonate, as it were, as one, I have an inkling of what this overriding reality is. And I have the taste in moments of the timeless actuality of this transcendent force. Madame even points out in her book that in that moment it is the soul itself that is present.

So please forgive me for, as it were, this repetition, but I need to be clear about the focus of my effort, the focus of this extraordinary work of dying to the known. What one doesn't see is one's slavery to the known. One does not see that this automaton is ceaselessly affirming itself. And I say "I" to every little affirmation, which is to be totally misguided. I wish to be empty. I'm reminded how the Dalai Lama said to one of our colleagues up in Toronto, that emptiness is consciousness. So I drop these pathetic affirmations that come from the automaton and I try to stay in front of—present to—that which is transcendent.

So one must die to the known in order for the unknown to be revealed. And the unknown is literally unknown. I guard against all of these petty inner arguments that I indulge in, to establish that I am privileged to point the way—things like that. The truth is I'm here to serve, to serve a very great and largely unknown purpose. I'm here, created in the image of God, to become as God, to be *deified*, as the theologians say. So I guard this emptiness; I wish to live in emptiness. And I need what is so rare in my own experience, in our experience: a state without tension.

And so I simply try *to be*. And I try to open to this extraordinary recognition of the timeless actuality of what is real, of what is transcendent. And through that, I begin to know the Self, that which is. And as Mme de Salzmann points out, to know the Self in me, to have this inkling in moments, is to be the Self. And through that I begin to acknowledge that this *be-ing* is without beginning or end—it is nothing that any of us creates. Rather, we open to its presence. And one begins to see that unless the parts come together, unless there's a new inner relation, I cannot open, I cannot be connected to Presence. I can't come to that through one brain or two, I need them all to be related. I need to open to the resonance in me of that which is.

So I try to keep the sense of tranquility, of becoming purified, of becoming whole. And I open to this world that lies beyond the literal constructs of the mind, and beyond this voracious egotism, and beyond all my avidity. And it is only through this work of purification that I can open to the workings of the ultimate life force. In the meantime, I work to be receptive to its action.

So this is a work that we share, that we explore together. And one needs to have a sense, as we go into manifestation and movement, that we are servants, we are here to serve this unknown. And so in a moment we should stop, and as I said go into manifestation still carrying this sense, this sense of a transcendent reality and a purpose to our lives. So let us stop.

# March 29, 2019—
# This Is a Work for Being

Those of you who have worked with me in this format know that I rarely have a script. At the same time, I should remind you that that which we are in search of—the Self with a capital S—belongs to the Absolute. It is no cheap thing, nothing I can buy on the supermarket shelf. At the same time, there are any number of extraordinary ways of entering into this search. And Mr. Gurdjieff, and Madame de Salzmann in turn, have been very clear about the terms on which this inquiry can be conducted.

Mr. Gurdjieff, in bringing these questions to the groups with which he worked, was very insistent on observing very clear terms of engagement. In any event, when we come here it is not to impose, or to get, or to manipulate, but it is to observe certain very exacting terms of (as it were) engagement.

And it begins with being in question. Who am I? What am I? Where am I? Mr. Gurdjieff was equally insistent, as Madame de Salzmann was, that we be honest. Because we can't come to anything real otherwise. Beginning right now. Because we are in search of Being. This is a work for Being. And we've been given this gift of life to serve. And it's not my ambitions that I serve; it's to serve a very, very high purpose. As I've reminded us on many an occasion, we've been created in the image of the Creator. And we are here to harken to an inner call. Madame refers to the nostalgia—which is not a sentimental thing: it is a real force in us, reminding us, calling us, to serve. And one must begin by becoming whole.

What we discover when we really observe is that we are fragmented. And so the first undertaking is to establish, as it were, a new order between the parts: between the head, the body, the feeling. And this is no cheap thing, no cheap undertaking. So this questioning opens me to the nature of this lack of order.

We might put it that we have three brains, and they are at odds with one another. So I need to find a way to enter into this inquiry that would enable a new order to appear. And as I quieten, and as I begin to settle, as it were, into this body, here in this moment—it's here in this moment because there is no time, there is only this moment—I can begin to listen to the resonance in me; in the mind, in the body, in the feeling; listen to the resonance of *I Am* in these parts. And one is immediately in touch with a fundamentally central aspect of this extraordinary teaching. Because as I quieten and as I collect my energies, I get an inkling that this central energy acts in my parts, and it acts as *I Am*. And I wish to open to that understanding—that the Self acts in me as I open to it.

And I begin to see that to know the Self is to be the Self. And I realize that there is Being in the scheme of things which is without beginning or end. So this is nothing to do with my subjectivity, my ambitions, my lust for power. On the contrary, it is to open to that which is real, to that which is transcendent. This is extraordinary material, and I get this inkling then of the timeless actuality of that which is transcendent. It is outside of time.

I see then that I need to work to be emptied of all my usual stuff—of my ferocious egoism, for one thing. Because that which is real is void of the ego. And I don't see that I am a slave of the ego. I'm a slave of this automatic and mechanical nature, which almost ceaselessly affirms itself. And I say "I" to every affirmation. But that is a dream, and I'm a slave, a prisoner, of that dream. And I need to begin to acknowledge and recognize this slavery.

So one's primary work is then to be in question. And one tries to listen to the resonance in oneself of *I Am*. As Madame points out, it is the soul itself that is here when I hear that resonance. The soul. And I betray this cosmic purpose to my creation if I blindly serve only my egoism and my dreams. So I see how important my posture is. I need to be erect. Because every kind of mutation, every kink in the neck or sloppiness in my posture affects the energy. So I try to be totally still and totally relaxed throughout. I try not to conduct a dialog inside, because I wish to open to a reality which is beyond the constructs of my usual mind, my usual thoughts. I wish to live in emptiness. And as the Dalai Lama has said, "Emptiness is consciousness." So one sees what an extraordinary obligation we are under through this gift of life.

I try not to be taken by these turning thoughts that surface and insinuate themselves, and I begin to acknowledge this requirement to be innerly silent, to be able, as it were, to pray without ceasing. And I begin to see and to listen to this resonance in me of *I Am*. It is a very real and very deep thing. And only when these parts—the head, the body, the feeling—come together and resonate as one, and not in contention with each other. It is only then that I can open to what is higher, open to Presence. This is such an extraordinary gift.

As Madame has pointed out, there is a cosmic need for this resonance, for these parts to resonate as one. And as I've said, it is no cheap thing to be in service of this ultimate call. Because I am here to serve, to serve a very high purpose. Even though one begins to sense that one's cosmic abode, the planet itself, is under extraordinary pressure itself, one must work regardless.

But again, check your postures, the set of your head. Every little tension upsets the equilibrium. And I begin to see I need a center of gravity for the attention. Otherwise I'm a slave of every prompting in me, every odd sensation, feeling, thought. I need a center of gravity. Mr. Gurdjieff is very clear that it is in the lower abdomen, where he says the astral body is connected to the physical body. And as I gather my thought, my energies, I see that this is a sound basis, a sound foundation for the possibility of a real I as opposed to this anemic, mechanical posturing that I flaunt. I need to acknowledge this extraordinary gift that Mr. Gurdjieff has given. And I need to keep this sobering look.

And when we go into action and we leave this format, try to keep some sense of that which is real, of that which is transcendent, of that which has a timeless actuality in my life. Because I'm here to serve. I'm not here to get, or to take, or destroy.

So now, very intentionally, I let this be. I still sustain this sense in me that *I Am*. And I try to carry that into my manifestation, as a service. And I try to remember what Madame has said, that "There is no time, only the present moment." And to carry that into my manifestation. So let us stop.

# April 9, 2019—
# There Is No Time

Strangely, since most of us, or I, haven't met most of you during my time [in the Foundation], it struck me I might safely begin with a few admonitions. And especially since I don't have a scripted text. So we will all, I trust, enter into this inquiry in the moment, together.

We are not here to get anything, or to achieve, or to boost our subjectivities. On that particular topic, let me say, or at least remind you as well as myself, of an occasion about thirty, forty years ago in which I described to Madame de Salzmann an experience I had had and she said to me, "That is Real I." And on the basis of that and subsequent explorations, I can assure you that Real I is void of the ego, void in fact of ethnicity. And this is really why we come. I come in order to open to the real, to the timeless actuality of that which is transcendent. Or to put it differently—again in Madame's and Gurdjieff's words—the Self, with a capital S, belongs to the Absolute. It is not a cheap thing.

Indeed, Gurdjieff reminds us that in order to investigate properly we need to approach this exploration with an all-centered balanced-being perceptiveness. Which again is not a cheap thing, and needs to be worked for. And so one sort of preliminary admonition might be to remind you, and myself, that we are ordinarily slaves, slaves of this automaton. And it is this that we need to become acquainted with and, as it were, to undermine.

Again, as Gurdjieff reminds us, the Self belongs to the Absolute. A very deep thing. And how does one come to see that, understand that? Madame put it so beautifully: that our work, what we undertake here now, together, is to die to the known. To die to the known in order to enter the unknown. So one needs to be reminded, as we are now, that "there is no time, only the present moment." That's not an invention of mine, those are Madame de Salzmann's words. And I see then that what I wish to open to is the timeless actuality of that which is transcendent. It is nothing that I invent; it created me, you, us all. And we've been given this extraordinary gift of life in order to serve that which is. In order to enable it to act in me. And it is at this point then that one begins to recognize the centrality of this concept and the reality of *I Am*.

And in order to come to that, I need to observe certain indications given by Mr. Gurdjieff. When we come here in this form, we need to work to be whole. What we've discovered is that we are fragmented, we are in parts. And Gurdjieff gives very strict indications of how to enter into that investigation, how to discover that I have three brains—this head, the body, the feeling. And what we all—I am sure—have discovered in our work in the quiet, as now, is that the *I Am* can resonate in me. It is nothing that I create, but rather, that I open to. For that, I need to be totally still, open, relaxed, erect, level-headed. A kink in the head, a tension in the spine, affects the energy. But Gurdjieff tells us to collect our thoughts. Those are his words "collect your thoughts." And that begins with the question: Who am I?

I've told you in other sittings the story of Moses, who had spoken to the burning bush, which had advised him to return to the Israelites. And he said, "Who shall I say hath sent me?" And the voice in the bush had said, "Say that *I Am* hath sent thee." And in moments I hear the resonance in me of *I Am*. As it sounds in me, these are three separate brains. It's only when these parts come into relation that I can be in touch with Presence. It is evidently not something available to one brain. It requires all the parts to resonate as one.

So this is a very deep work. And I try to listen wordlessly. I'm not here to justify my subjectivity, and why I want this and don't like that. Because that is done mechanically. The automaton affirms itself at every turn, and to each affirmation I blindly say "I, I, I." And we must see this slavery, we must see this betrayal of the higher through our stupidity, our arrogance, our sleep. I must trust the silence and I must stand unknowing in that presence. I accept to be emptied. A friend in Toronto reminded me that his friend, the Dalai Lama, had said to him, "Emptiness is consciousness." I need to open myself to this emptiness; I need to live in emptiness. And there come these moments when, in silence, I can open to energies in me that have not yet taken a form—of a dream, or egoism.

And I am reminded of how Mr. Gurdjieff respected these transcendent indications of what it is to be a real human being. Indeed he said in one meeting, "You are not tail of donkey." And he explained how each of us has a role to play in repairing the past, a role to play in what he called the line of one's blood. This is a far cry from the arrogant selfishness that we tend to display. So I try to be whole, open, accepting of the extraordinary mystery of being given this gift of life. The great traditions say that the aim of human life is God-realization, to become as God. Which in itself is an extraordinary search to undertake.

And so one begins to sense that we've been given life in order to serve, not just to get and to take and to trample on. And then one sees in moments, one has this inkling of a higher power. So one should take seriously these indications that we are indeed slaves of this automaton, and that we don't see it. And that is really an overriding demand. One measures one's sleep against such moments in which one sees this slavery, in which one recognizes what Gurdjieff calls this ferocious egotism that grabs convulsively. And there it is, staring us in our faces, the work that needs to be done to wake up, to begin consciously to occupy this body, this instrument. It's an extraordinary gift, this life.

Even now I must watch my posture. I need a real purification. And I see that I need a center of gravity for the attention, otherwise it is constantly taken, betrayed. Remember that you are not tail of donkey. And remember too that there is no time. I'm quoting: there is only the present moment. And I need to savor that present moment. It is in this present moment that I find myself on the Way.

So it is so good and so right that we come together in this form, to enter into the silence which is at the very source of our lives. And we have Gurdjieff's extraordinary indication to support this search, that "Life is real only then, when 'I Am.'" Extra-ordinary. "Life is real only then, when 'I Am.'" So there's so much to be understood and to be taken in. One has a being-duty to serve.

So now as we ready ourselves to go into movement, let us try to keep this thread, this sense of *I Am*. Try to keep it intact, and not just for five minutes, but again, and again. And one recognizes then that this is such an extraordinary teaching. And it isn't for slaves, it is for those who wish to have being, real life.

So let us finish. And when we clear the room, to do it with intention, as a service.

# May 3, 2019—
# There Is No Death

I do not have a formal presentation, as it were, and so I will begin with a deep recollection that I had of being in the house at Mendham sixty-odd years ago, on the evening on which Madame Ouspensky passed away. I recall being given the opportunity to go into her room, which I'd never done until then, to see her.

What I'm leading up to is that two days later we received this extraordinary letter from Madame de Salzmann in which she pointed out—and I quote—"There is no death, life cannot die." And coming from her, this was an almost, as it were, historic declaration. Decades later, I discovered that the editors of her book had rather arbitrarily put that passage in the middle of an undistinguished section in the middle of the book of her talks and teaching. And I suppose our work is to unearth and acknowledge these extraordinary insights.

We might begin today with any one of any number of extraordinary indications given to us by Mr. Gurdjieff and Madame de Salzmann. I've brought one of those indications a number of times, so it might not hurt to hear yet again that we are here, and our work is "to die to the known." And one dies to the known in order to enter the unknown. How to meet that encompassing directive? Here, now? And so one sees that one needs once again to make the effort, the attempt, to situate oneself in the present. Again, Madame has pointed out that there is no time, only the present moment.

And Mr. Gurdjieff himself, if one studies the accounts of his meetings, is very clear on how one enters into this exploration. Because the aim in coming together like this and exploring like this is in order to meet Mr. Gurdjieff's and Madame's direction that we try to become whole. And so my effort is to establish quietly that I am indeed a three-brained entity—with a head, body, and feelings. And so I need to find myself in the present moment, in this body, with a mind that isn't wandering off into memories or fantastic dreams. Because it is here, in the present moment, that I can learn that life does not die. And it calls for a great emphasis in the direction that Mr. Gurdjieff indicated. He used these words: "To gather one's thoughts." His words.

And so it's very important to guard my posture, to be vertical, to be grounded in the body. And, as it were, to put myself in question: Who am I? Who indeed am I? I need to be relaxed, without tension, and cognizant of the fact that as I relax and become purified in all these parts, I actually open to the timeless actuality of what is real, of what is transcendent. And so in moments I listen, as Madame put it, I listen to the resonance in me of *I Am*. And again this *I Am* is nothing that I pick up in the gutter or something that I invent. It is. It is before I was. And this *I Am*, which is of a different scale, a different cosmic scale, can resonate in these, if you wish, brains.

And what is important then in such a moment is what Madame points out, that the soul itself is present. The soul itself. And the soul is a very high thing. It's not something I buy in the supermarket. And there come these moments in which I can in fact know the soul. Moments. And again as Madame has put it, to know the soul is to be the soul. Such extraordinary material—if we are open, if I am without tension, if I am not dreaming.

This is such a demanding undertaking. And it is only when these parts come together that I truly open to presence. Presence cannot be known through one center only. It can be known only through what Gurdjieff refers to as "all-brained balanced-being perceptiveness." It is not a cheap thing. All-brained balanced-being perceptiveness. And truly, it is only through that that I can die to the known, to all I am attached to. And I'm attached to very coarse and base phenomena.

So I try to be relaxed, open. As Meister Eckhart puts it, one must trust in abandonment, letting go. Letting go. And so I can follow the breath, and as I breathe in, I can say "I," and as I breathe out, "Am." And Gurdjieff, as I've mentioned, says that when I breathe in, it's as if something stands up inside. And when I breathe out, it's as if something sits down. And I see that I don't really stay too long; I don't stay connected too long. And yet the breath brings the life. And he says I'm part of a great being that breathes and gives me life. I need to know this and acknowledge this, this extraordinary gift of life.

Madame, in turn, has pointed out that I need to come to a sensation of the void. And so it is not untimely to be reminded that we are here to serve. And to be reminded, as I've tried to do, that I wish to be free of the egoism. As Madame has pointed out, we are slaves of the automatism, which is ceaselessly affirming itself. And to every affirmation I say "I"—"I" this, "I" that. And that's really a betrayal of the very extraordinary knowledge contained in this teaching.

And as I've reminded us again, I recall bringing to Madame de Salzmann an account of an extraordinary experience. And she had said to me, "That is Real I." And on the basis of that and further explorations down the years I can faithfully declare that Real I is void of the ego. And our work is to be detached, to abandon the ego. Because the Self is what is real, and it belongs to the Absolute. And we have inklings in moments of the timeless actuality of that which is the source.

So try to sustain a certain sense of purity and of wholeness here, now. Indeed, there is that in us which has a nostalgia for this reality. It's not a petty, emotional thing, it is a longing to be whole, real, balanced. A longing for presence. And so one must see the workings in us of our ferocious egoisms, and to try not to identify, not to be slaves. And one sees that when one opens to that which is real, one is not alone. And one sees that there are these moments where "I," "I," "I," opens to *I Am*. That the *I Am* resonates without my interference, without my "doing."

So try to sustain this sense of the transcendent. And try, when we go into movement, and into manifestation, to have some contact with the reality that is ordinarily hidden. And as I've reminded us at the start, life cannot die. There is no death. Can we try to be faithful to that understanding? And so, can we make a kind of seamless transition into movement and manifestation in the way we put the chairs away?

So let us stop.

# June 11, 2019—
# To Pay for My Arising

I think it is worth being reminded that when we come together like this in this format, it is not to *get* anything, not to *achieve* anything. And we can't go or come closer to our approach in this teaching at this time than to be reminded of what Madame de Salzmann has said—that we are here to "die to the known." And we die to the known, as possible, in order to enter the unknown, in order to open to that which is real.

Mr. Gurdjieff was very precise in his entry into this exploration. And Madame de Salzmann was also very clear in indicating that in this exploration, there is no time, only the present moment. How then to enter into this exploration, on those terms? Gurdjieff, in his extraordinary way, indicated the need for all-centered balanced-being perceptiveness. And that isn't a given, it has to be earned.

So one takes seriously this need—to begin, as Mr. Gurdjieff indicates, by actually asking, "Who am I?" He said that one must gather one's thoughts. He said it—to gather one's thoughts. Each of us can enter into that investigation for himself or herself. After all, I am allegedly a three-brained being. I have a head brain, this body brain, and the feeling. And I can quietly, silently, wordlessly, try to establish in some way that I am indeed three-brained. I *know* that I am here, I *sense* through the body that I am here, and I open to the *feeling*. I see too that I need to watch my posture. If I'm bent, angled, crooked, what kind of energy corresponds? Really nothing that I am interested in. And I trust the silence. I don't fill the space with my inner talking and my dreams and my imagination. I wish to be emptied. And as I've reminded us, the Dalai Lama has pointed out that emptiness is consciousness. And one needs to open to indications, inklings, that this is indeed so. And it is indeed so when one begins to open to the resonance in oneself of the *I Am*.

The *I Am* is very central to this extraordinary teaching. It is nothing that I invent; it is. And as I quieten and as a new order begins to take shape in me and through me, wordlessly, I receive this inkling that the *I Am* manifests in each of the parts. And it resonates equally in the parts.

The strange thing is that this exploration is ongoing, and has been, down the centuries. I was reading an extremely interesting account of the hesychast tradition in eastern orthodoxy by a hesychast bishop [Kallistos Ware] who lives in the British Isles. And he has pointed out how the hesychasts, the monks, and of course how the nuns, have come to this realization of the need to be in the presence of God, and to be praying. But the prayer is not to get, and, the bishop points out, it is not the monk who is making the declaration. To him, it is the creator himself who prays in us. What an extraordinary thought, and completely in correspondence with what Mr. Gurdjieff brings. So it is not this little personage who is praying—it is the creator himself who brings his prayer.

And in moments, too, we have this inkling of the actuality of the higher, of the divine. And that we've been created in the image of God. We have this from all of the great revelations—we have been created in the image of God, to serve a very great purpose.

As I've said, it is not to get or to achieve or to pander to my egoism. Indeed, that which is real is void of the ego. It is void too, in fact, of ethnicity. I remember reporting to Madame de Salzmann—forty, fifty years ago—an experience in a local church in Grand Central Station and later out on Fifth Avenue, in which I was totally free. And she said to me, "That is Real I." On the basis of that, and decades of exploration, I can assure you that Real I is indeed void of the ego. And so one sees that there is a real life beyond the formulations of the thought. And I must open to that reality. It is not so much my birthright as my duty to pay for my arising.

And so it isn't untimely to be reminded that in our teaching we humans in our sleep are really slaves of the automaton. I walk around imagining that I am awake, but I am a slave to this automaton, which is ceaselessly affirming itself through its dreams, associations, tensions, negativity. And to each of these affirmations I say "I," "I." But that is the farthest thing from the I. It is our duty to attempt, as seriously as we can, not to be slaves, not to obey these automatic affirmations. And so in moments one opens to the resonance in one of the *I Am*. And as Madame points out, when there is this resonance in me of that which is real, I have this inkling, this taste, of the Self. Madame de Salzmann says that the soul itself is present in such a moment—the soul itself, which is a very high thing. It speaks of the essential, of the Real, of the transcendent. So I try to be totally centered, open, listening.

One sees then that what one really wishes is to return to the source. In moments one sees the Self—with a capital S—in moments. And when one sees the Self—and I quote Madame de Salzmann—"I am the Self."

So one sees that these sittings open one to that which is real, which can be met only wordlessly, respectfully. One begins truly to sense that we are here to serve a very great purpose, and that purpose can't be served unless I consciously enter into this exploration. And I serve by guarding the attention, this special force. So I try to follow the breath; I would not be here without the breath, and I can intentionally breathe in. And Gurdjieff even says that when I breathe in, it's as if something stands up in me, and when I breathe out, it's as if something sits down in me. And one begins to see that I am *being breathed.*

And so I then undertake, as much as possible, not to be a slave of this automaton, not to be driven by this shallow egotism, but to try to value and carry this sense of the transcendent, even as I walk in the street, as I roll up a carpet. And I try to work, as all of the great revelations indicate, for my deification. Which is another way of saying that I wish to become as God. And I see it as my duty.

So let us intentionally end this inner exploration and go into manifestation like conscious beings.

# September 20, 2019—We Are in God

It is good that we come together like this. I must confess that I do not have a prepared script or text, but I did think to take the risk of reading two extraordinary thoughts that have emerged in the, as it were, orthodox teachings of the proponents and explorers from which Mr. Gurdjieff emerged. And the first is: "When you pray, you yourself must be silent. Let the prayer speak." And a corresponding thought from this deep exploration of the same religious sources from which our teaching has sprung, that "True inner prayer is to stop talking and to listen to the wordless voice of God within our hearts."

And so really that is what we ourselves explore when we come together to what we call work. Because even in this building, we forget that we are ordinarily slaves of the automatism. And we do not recognize enough that it is this automatism which ceaselessly affirms itself. And to each affirmation one says "I." One says "I like, I am, I want, I wish, I can, I can't," and this is a kind of a plague. And one has this impression that we do not adequately acknowledge this awesome burden.

After all, as Mr. Gurdjieff reminds us, we are created in the image of God. And our aim is to open to the timeless actuality of the transcendent in us, and we do not see that we ignore that actuality. And this is not a small or cheap thing. If you remember that at Christmas 1948 Mr. Gurdjieff gave his exercise. And he urged the audience—our forebears, as it were—to use this indication, not to ape anything, not to pretend. Instead he said "Become Christ. Be." He did not say become *like* Christ: rather, *become* Christ. And so this is what we need to focus on. And so, we need to listen—deeply, exactly—to the wordless voice of God that is in our hearts. And as I've said, this is no cheap thing, not a cheap exercise. For that work, I need to find myself in the presence of God, without pretending or faking, but to acknowledge the obstacles, to acknowledge one's slavery to what is mechanical, automatic, subconscious. And so I need to be silent inwardly in order to be open, sensitive, attentive. Because, and again to repeat myself, Madame put it so brilliantly: that we need to die to the known, in order to enter the unknown. And I need to face that now, wordlessly. I need to be still.

Mr. Gurdjieff emphasizes this necessity, and he emphasizes the need to enter into this search in a special way. And this special way is to bring order in myself. I need to ask, Who am I? And I need to take Mr. Gurdjieff at his word, that I am created a three-brained being. And I verify now that I have a mind; a body in which I am situated, vertically, unmoving; and I have a feeling nature. We say rather loosely that it is situated in the heart. And without arguing or playing my little inner games, I try to take in these impressions. Because my aim is to become whole. And to die to the known, to all that I assume is real, including, and especially, my subjectivity. Because the truth is that Real I is void of the ego. How to work towards that?

So in a profound sense then, I wish to appear, to stand, in the presence of God. And one sees how extraordinarily informative Mr. Gurdjieff's teaching is, in this respect. And how exceptionally accurate his great injunction to us is, that "Life is real only then, when *I Am*." And you remember this famous event about the burning bush: when Moses was asked to return to his people, he asked this burning bush, "Who shall I say hath sent me?" And the voice in the bush said, "Say that *I Am* hath sent thee." The *I Am* is so absolutely central to Mr. Gurdjieff's teaching. When I am still, quiet, receptive, I experience these moments, this inkling that *I Am* enters my parts. And it enters my parts and conveys a sense of presence only when I am whole. That sense of being whole does not come just as I want it or wish it; it has to be earned.

And so again as Madame has put it so concisely, one begins to verify that there is no time, only the present moment. And I wish to be in the present moment, actually. And so one begins to see, as these long-term students of the practice of the presence of God discover, that to pray is to stand before God, to know that we are in God and He is in us.

So I begin to sense the demand. As I've said, it is not a cheap thing. Then one discovers that it is not only I who pray, but that it is God himself who calls to me. We are blinded to this by our mechanicality, by our arrogance, by our egotism. What a privilege then it is to work with you, with others, in order to open to what is real. Madame has said also, I am already that which I seek to be. And so my work is to purify my effort, to learn how to pray, how to stand in the presence of God, who is also in me. And I try to occupy the body, to feel myself erect, in contact with the earth. And open to the timeless actuality of the transcendent—or if you wish, of God. So it's an extraordinary privilege to have been created a human being.

So one tries to remain attentive to the resonance in me of *I Am*, because it is such a central aspect of the Gurdjieff teaching. And to be reminded then that Life is Real only then, when *I Am*. It's nothing to do with what I like, what I don't like. It is about a new objectivity, impartiality. And opening to what is real, opening to Presence.

And it's so strange that we can think and work to become real at this very moment, when one sees more of the extraordinary pressures arising on planet Earth. All the more reason to work, to pay for one's arising, to work for being.

And so, in a moment, let us leave this. But try to clear the room in a new way. So let us stop.

# October 18, 2019—
# The Need to Birth the Soul

Since we met last time, I ventured to suggest that we ponder some of the extraordinary thoughts that have emerged from centers like this in the old Middle East and other hesychast enclaves, and I'd like to bring these thoughts again at odd moments. But in the subsequent course of our explorations I rediscovered a thought of Mr. Gurdjieff's that he had brought back in 1922, and I will repeat it with the hope that we can discover some of the implications of what he brought.

Mr. Gurdjieff put this very bluntly, as it were, when he declared: "There is no evolution of the masses, only of individuals." And in the course of my research I've discovered that certain of our contemporaries—recent contemporaries—have fathomed some of the implications of a thought such as that, that there is no evolution of the masses, only of individuals.

I feel we've touched on these implications in the way that we have attempted to fathom the implications of what Mr. Gurdjieff has brought. We are, as it were, obliged to pursue these implications. Obliged, as I've reminded us, because Mr. Gurdjieff was very clear, very precise, in his indications. After all, in speaking through Madame de Salzmann, among others, he reminds us that we are ordinarily slaves of the automatism. And this automatism is endlessly affirming itself, automatically. And we in our blindness, and with our limited perspective, identify all the time with these automatic, egoistic affirmations. Because strangely, around us there are, as it were, many seekers of the truth, who are doing and attempting what Mr. Gurdjieff has brought to us: this need—and I use some awkward language—this need to birth the soul. And these days you hear around you the use of the word—and words like—*sophia*, which is wisdom, the truth, and we want to be nurtured by that. We wish to grow in that atmosphere.

So we have the need then to understand that we are learning how to pray, learning how to come into the presence of God. What we discover then is that we are not only, as it were, living in God, but that God lives in us. Extraordinary. It's not a one-sided exchange. When I am truly still, I open to the fact that I am created—as we are told—in the image of God. And through his wordless prayer, I learn that He is in me. And I know that through being still, silent.

What we call prayer is often just talking—talking to oneself, arguing one's case. And one doesn't see that this is sheer limitation and mere egoism. I can assure you from my own experience and Madame's indications to me—that Real I is void of the ego, void even of ethnicity. And I begin to discover that I need to become whole, to have a real relation between the head brain, the body, and the feeling. And this is no cheap thing, and it's no accident. It is something that I need to begin to open to, now. To meet it with what has been called a choiceless awareness.

And one is reminded again that when Mr. Gurdjieff brought this (as it were) Christmas 1948 direction, he said, "Become Christ. Be." He didn't say, become "like Christ." Rather, "Become Christ." We've begun to see the need to enter into this movement towards deification. Nothing less. Nothing less, because evolution is not for the masses. And I need to investigate, explore.

I see then this need for the purification of my efforts, of my thought. Because through this purification I open to this extraordinary movement, this extraordinary force that we know as "I Am" and which is so central to this teaching. And there come these moments when I have an inkling of this, when I open to the resonance in me of that which is real, transcendent. You may remember that last time we met, I quoted something which the folks on Mount Athos and hesychasts down the ages, and their compatriots living today, understand--that "When you pray, you yourself must be silent—let the prayer speak."

There was a second thought that I brought, from the same source, which is alive today, as exemplified by the work of Bishop Kallistos Ware in England, for example: "True inner prayer is to stop talking and to listen to the wordless voice of God within our hearts." So that we find that when we pray, when we stand in the presence of God, we know that *we are in God and that He is in us*. And so one finds evidence now that in our time some extraordinary beings on this beleaguered planet have come to see that this work to be a real individual leads up to an extraordinary work which is titled "individuation."

There is some extraordinary documentation of this. And so one must take Mr. Gurdjieff seriously when he counsels us to work with the *I Am*. As I've reminded us, we have this extraordinary story going back to the time of Moses, when the voice in the burning bush told him to return to his people, and he asked, "Who shall I say hath sent me?" The voice in the bush said, "Say that *I Am* hath sent thee." Again, when we work quietly and intensely and objectively, we have an inkling of what that means, that *I Am* enters one's parts. One opens to that which is timeless, the timeless actuality of the transcendent. Through this, I see that the true purpose of my life is to serve this Presence, and I can know it only through being whole, not by being in parts or pieces or dreaming.

And as Mr. Gurdjieff makes it so plain, one discovers that "Life is real only then, when *I Am.*" And strangely, this work is ever more needed when one takes in the evidence that our abode, the Earth, is under enormous cosmic pressures. My friend Peter Kingsley has sensed this as strongly as ever, and calls me from Mount Athos to exchange on that topic.

And so we also need to know, or open to, an understanding of the afterlife. Mr. Gurdjieff makes it clear that there is a whole, as it were, world of energies between our level and that of the Creator, filled with angels, archangels, cherubim, seraphim. And so there's another extraordinary realm in this teaching that needs to be very clearly examined and understood. I refer to the question, the topic of angelology. So there's so much to be explored and shared. I need to grow in that service. I am here to work for being. I'm not here to indulge all of my weaknesses, all of my subjectivity, which is at such a low level. And I referred to Peter Kingsley, whose latest book has the subtitle of "Carl Jung and the End of Humanity." If it is true, if these pressures are beyond our capacity to bear, we should be at least more and more sensitive. I said to Kingsley that I hope to make a seamless departure, and he said, "And the second time?" So there are so many unknowns, so many mysteries, which we need to face and acknowledge.

And so, without losing this sense of being more whole, of needing to work for being, of needing to serve the Creator, let us stop. But in leaving, to keep this effort active, as a duty, as a service. And recognizing, as much as one can, the need to grow, sensibly, sanely. So let us stop.

# November 8, 2019—
# I Am that I Am

I trust that you will, as you have in the past, bear with me because I do not have a script or a prepared text. But you will recall that last time we were together I quoted something that Mr. Gurdjieff had said back in 1922, that there is no evolution for the masses, only for the individual. And so each of us tries to come to the elusive state of all-centered balanced-being perceptiveness.

And from one profound perspective one may say that we are learning how to pray. How to appear—if you wish, how to stand—in the presence of God. Because it has been said, and the great revelations are in accord on this, that we have been created in the image of God. God is, of course, transcendent. And I wish to open to this transcendent actuality. I have to come to see and recognize and understand that He is in me, as I am in Him, listening to his wordless intimations. And in order to open to that actuality I need to be silent, still, in all my parts.

And as I've said so many times, Mr. Gurdjieff gave very, very precise indications of how to begin that investigation and to establish this relation. Because—again as I've reminded us all—we do not see our slavery to the automaton, to this entity, to this three-brained entity. And our first necessity is to work for unity. Because Presence can't be known simply through one part. So I need to wordlessly and silently come to this understanding, that the head and the body and the feeling need to come into a new alignment, into this all-centered relationship. It is not just a verbal undertaking; in fact, I must put my thoughts to rest, let them subside. And I open quietly, wordlessly, to the impression that I exist—which is in itself another mystery. Because at the very center of Mr. Gurdjieff's teaching is this understanding of the centrality of *I Am*. And I have these moments, these inklings, these intimations, that *I Am* occupies me. In fact *I Am that I Am*.

For that, I need to be so watchful and vigilant to the state that I find myself in. I need to be erect, level-headed, sensitive, accepting, and obedient. I allow this opening in me. And I begin to discern this resonance in me of *I Am*. And respect it. Because as Madame has pointed out so beautifully, the soul itself is present. The soul itself. And the soul belongs to the Absolute.

And one sees then why the practicing hesychasts such as Bishop Kallistos Ware point out that when you pray, you yourself must be silent—let the prayer speak. Do watch your posture. Be erect without tension, without any inner talking, without any argument, because as I've said, without the attention I am simply a slave of the automaton. And I don't see that it perpetually affirms itself, and I equally perpetually say "I" to its mechanical affirmations. I work then to trust the attention, and to ignore, discard the inner talk and the justification. One doesn't see the scope of the egoism. And we do not see that the purpose of our being created in the image of God is to serve Presence. We don't see what a disservice we perform when we, as it were, nurture only the egoism. And I've quoted to you Mr. Gurdjieff's instruction in that 1948 Christmas Day instruction that he gave. He said to work, and "Become Christ." He did not say be like Christ, or similar to Christ; he said—I quote—"Become Christ. Be." So this is a work for being, to serve a very, very great purpose. Unstintingly.

And you will remember that last time we met, I invoked the hereafter. Not just this present life, but the hereafter, which is largely a mystery. The hereafter, according to the developed ones, is populated with angels, archangels, cherubim, seraphim, and other entities. The hereafter is, from one perspective, the imaginal world. The imaginal world that Henry Corbin and Peter Kingsley and other advanced beings point us to. And I'm reminded that Madame puts it this way too: that the centers have to submit to a common master, and that when there is no master there is no soul—neither soul nor will. So these extreme obligations come with this human form and life that we've been given. And we are obligated to investigate, to examine, to explore, to question this extraordinary life that we have been given.

And as I've pointed out, too, as we look more closely and clearly at ourselves and our surroundings, we see that the planet too is under extraordinary pressures. But at the same time, we are duty-bound to work, to serve, come what may.

Mr. Gurdjieff was such an extraordinary being. And he reminded us also of so many things, including the work to repair the past. He said, in one of his talks, I believe it was to the people in Paris, that "You are not tail of donkey." That we have a role in repairing the past, the mistakes—even of our forebears, if you read that clearly. And so we come to see our obligations in moments when we have this inkling of the *I Am*, when we have this resonance in us of the Self. That when we have these inklings, we can sense the Self. One can *feel* the Self. And again as Madame has pointed out, that when I know the Self, I am the Self.

So there's such extraordinary and, as it were, miraculous movements that take place when I work to be whole and to acquire being. So we really need to respect the call that comes—that comes, as it were, through the voiceless call, the voiceless urging of the Creator. And I should work to appear more often in His presence, remembering that it isn't just through thought, just through feeling, or just through some movement. It has to be the whole being. All-centered.

And so perhaps, then, we should stop, but not to forget. Not just to be wrapped up in one's imagination, one's dream, in one's ferocious egoism, as Madame put it—one's ferocious egoism.

And so let us stop. At the same time, keeping contact with this inner reality, remembering that there is this life force at work, and I'm here to serve it. So thank you for being here and wishing to serve.

# December 13, 2019—
# The Right to Serve

I have to confess that the quality of the work here among those who have been regular has been so extraordinarily deep that I haven't, as it were, prepared a script, but rather approach this moment as being totally unknown.

We might even simply take up one of the extraordinary thoughts that Mr. Gurdjieff and Madame de Salzmann have brought—for example, we might explore what it means "to die to the known." And one tries to die to the known in order that the unknown can act.

I'm telling you nothing you don't know when I say that Mr. Gurdjieff was very clear and insistent on the way one enters into a work such as we are undertaking as I speak. And he was insistent that we begin by establishing a unity between our parts, that we become whole. Because this work isn't about grabbing, getting. It is about earning the right to serve, to serve the creator. And even as we come to that thought, one must acknowledge that one is part of God and that God is in me—wordlessly calling to each of us, severally and as a group, to serve, to serve the transcendent.

And really, no matter where one begins, one begins to see the truth of his great guiding thought: that life is real only then, when *I Am*. And as I've reminded you, often, *I Am* is a very central element of Mr. Gurdjieff's teaching. One can go back to the time of Moses, if you wish, to get a reading on that. It had to do with the voice in the burning bush that told Moses to go back to his people. Moses said, "Who shall I say hath sent me?" And the voice in the burning bush said, "Say that *I Am* hath sent thee."

And can you link with this in any way as I mention it? Because our work is to live this teaching, to exemplify the attention in my posture, in my words, in my feeling. I do not have to invent some overriding theory. We have been given and we have received these extraordinary indications. And the *I Am* isn't something one invents—it is; it is before I was. To savor this I need to be totally in the present, not arguing with myself, not talking about getting something, not looking at the clock to wonder how soon I can get out, because I must learn how to serve. I have been created in the image of God in order to serve. And in order to serve I need to have being, I work for being. Not to give orders, to push people about, to get something for nothing. I am here to pay for my arising. Can I feel that, now?

And then one realizes that I work to stand in the presence of God. And when I stand in the presence of God I pray, I can pray. As some latterday hesychast has put it in our own time, "To pray is to stand before God, to know that we are in God and He is in us." And these hesychasts who have worked in the lineage of Mr. Gurdjieff understand that "When you pray, you yourself must be silent, let the prayer speak."

So, as my sense of being whole grows, I have inklings that the *I Am* is acting in me—in the head brain, in the body, in the feeling. I slowly have this inkling, this taste, of the resonance in me of *I Am*. I don't try and fake it or make it happen or argue about it. I try to be open, contained, whole, balanced. And I see that my work is to echo the understanding of the Creator. As I open to this resonance in me of *I Am*, I can sense Presence. I sense the transcendent. I don't invent or fake; I wish to serve. I see then that my posture is so important—my verticality, my levelheadedness, my containment, my whole valuation of who I am. I'm not here to give orders, to take, to push people around. I am here to serve. So I see that my aim is in fact deification. As they say in the traditions, to be as God.

But Mr. Gurdjieff went further when he gave his famous Christmas exercise. He told people: "Become Christ. Be." He didn't say become like Christ, he said "Become Christ." This is extraordinary knowledge—that we are on the planet to serve. And as Mr. Gurdjieff and Madame tell us, there is a cosmic need for the being that I would wish to be. A cosmic need.

And even now I might risk a subtle warning since I've mentioned the cosmic aspect. As I said in the toast on January 13th—I slipped it in at the end—the earth itself is under pressure. We look at all of the signs of global warming and other, as it were, natural disasters. So we have a work, to work with purity and sincerity and an integrity. Otherwise we are simply slaves, as Mr. Gurdjieff said, of the automatism which ceaselessly affirms its subjectivity, its likes and dislikes. These affirmations are purely mechanical. And I say "I," "I" to every one of them because I have no attention, no discrimination.

So even now, have some taste of an inner life which includes the breathing. I'm here because I breathe, I'm able to be here because I can breathe. And slowly one has this inkling of Presence, as the parts resonate as one. I have the taste of Self. And merely to taste the Self is to know the Self. This is Gurdjieff talking—not me.

And I thought you might like to hear something that Mr. Gurdjieff said on May 16, 1942. He said: "On earth millions of human beings pray. All of their prayers produce a particular substance, and owing to the law that substances with the same affinities tend to join, to accumulate in one place, the substance produced by prayers accumulates in certain places in space, and then at a single point through contact with that point. The force that accumulates there is even great enough to form an individual. Now, one can take this substance and accumulate it in oneself."

And so I try to listen to the resonance in myself of *I Am*. This effort is not something I do once a month, while in the meantime I talk and jabber and carry on like a person possessed. I see that I have to clean up my act, my inner act. And so, wordlessly, with an active inner attention, I open to this new sense of Presence. I see that the sense of Presence can be known only when I am unified. It's not available to me simply through the thought or body tension or some stray feeling. It is an all-brained balanced-being perception, which are Mr. Gurdjieff's words. And he called us again and again and again to explore this possibility. To explore this cosmic need.

And I thought I would quote the words of an old friend, Swami Jyotirmayananda, an Indian swami who actually visited us at Mendham, and came to the Foundation one day. And when he writes or greets people like you and me, his manner of addressing us is to say, "Blessed Self, adorations." Blessed Self. This is what we need to explore—the life within this Blessed Self that each of us is. So can we carry this intensity, this inner intensity—can we carry this live attention into our activities, into putting the chairs away, into going out into life? Because this is why Mr. Gurdjieff brought the teaching and made his sacrifices. And why a generation or two who are no longer with us worked to grow their being.

So can we now very intentionally go into movement, into manifestation, while remembering. And to those of you who have been so regular and faithful, thank you: we share something.

# January 31, 2020—
# The Sense of Verticality

I am more or less at a loss as to an appropriate introduction, especially since you've been so diligent in sharing the particular approach that we have followed. And yet the real aim of coming together is to be silent. Indeed, as the hesychasts and our forebear's advise us, we need to be silent in our prayer. And if I may risk total misunderstanding, I believe that we come here in order to stand in the presence of the Creator and to pray.

And how does one stand in the presence of the transcendent, of that which is, that which was before we were born? Mr. Gurdjieff was so clear in his indications, in his instructions that there is a real, as it were, procedure to be followed when we meet as we do. He has said very clearly that one must begin this work by establishing an inner order. I see—and I'm sure you agree—that it is an absolute necessity to work as three-brained entities, not just in the thought or through some reaction in the body or some automatic emotional persuasion. But to try to be whole.

So I see this demand to become whole, and I enter that wordlessly—not arguing with "me" and "mine" about what "I" like or don't like, but to be still. Because, in the first place, we are created, it is said, in the image of God. I am IN God, and God is IN me. I don't argue about it. And I wish to meet this work for being in silence. It is an extraordinary demand. We have been created in order to meet that high purpose. And that purpose is not to gratify *me* and *mine*. I'm not here to get anything.

I sense now something of the reason for being created as we are. It has to do with serving a very high purpose. As Madame de Salzmann put it, "there is a cosmic need for the being that I would wish to be." A cosmic need. So I need to approach this extraordinary inner search as a duty.

Again as I've said, I'm not here to get, but I'm here to serve. And even now, at this point, I begin to sense some of the extraordinary implications and consequences. One extraordinary unfolding is reaching one even now, and that has to do with the centrality of *I Am*—a very central component, as it were, of Mr. Gurdjieff's teaching. And slowly as I enter the silence, I receive this intimation, this inkling, as it were, of that extraordinary aspect of life. Wordlessly, in the silence. Beyond the basic constructs of the mind. And if I work for being, it is not through the ego.

Slowly something begins to inch its way into this conglomerate that I am, this three-brained entity. You must forgive my hesitation, but one sees the extraordinary difficulty, the enormity of the undertaking, to become whole. And it is only through that that I can open to the presence in me of *I Am*. Slowly *I Am* begins to filter in. It begins to resonate in me. And that is an extraordinary process. Because in that resonance the soul itself is known, which in itself is a profound unfolding. And as Mr. Gurdjieff has indicated, the *I Am* is a very essential, central, fundamental aspect of the human being. It becomes known only through this invisible inner struggle to be whole. And I need to be still, silent, accepting, purified, in order to participate in that unfolding.

So one discovers why Mr. Gurdjieff, as it were, let a deep secret out of the bag when he said that "Life is real only then, when *I Am*." It isn't real when I'm telling myself all these stories about *me* and *mine*. As I've told you, Madame put it to me one day in such a clear way that I could tell, once and for all, that Real I is void of the ego. And so one respects this work to be whole. Forgive me for all of this seeming hesitancy, but this is such a profound and extraordinary work. It is a very moving impression when we share this effort, when we find ourselves, as it were, standing in the presence of the Creator, in the presence of that which is transcendent.

And it is an especially deep exploration at a time like the present, when the planet itself is under pressure. One must work with a profound impartiality. This knowledge is no cheap thing, in fact it has to be paid for by one's effort, the effort to respect the silence, and the verticality, of our being. And in the course of this, one almost forgets to emphasize so many aspects of that work for being.

Let me quote this extraordinary line that I found in Madame's book: "The wish to be conscious is the wish to be. It can only be understood in silence." And as I've repeatedly reminded us all, we are ordinarily slaves of the automatism, the automaton, this entity, which is endlessly affirming its presence, its reaction, its contrarian wish, its wish to pay nothing. So try to be, as it were, unmoving, whole, because through that one is paying for one's arising. And work such as we're attempting now is a need, it is needed in the scheme of things.

So can I verify—quietly, without moving, without any inner talk—can I verify this sense of verticality, the sense that *I Am*. When we leave and go into manifestation, can we try to keep some sense of and connection with this reality. There are so many exercises and indications that we should try to take up—like working with the breath, working to have a center of gravity. Always as something actual and not just verbal. And so then, can I keep this orientation to *I Am*.

Now let us stop.

# February 21, 2020—Opening to Presence

I thought to bring us together, as it were, by quoting something that Madame de Salzmann reminded us of—that the wish to be conscious is the wish to be. And she emphasized that this is something that can only be understood in silence.

I'm reminded in turn to forego any secondary thought, while we explore the thought that I just put out. And as I've mentioned a number of times, the practice in the traditional centers such as those of the hesychasts, those on Mount Athos, and the people around Mr. Gurdjieff, was to declare that our questioning needs to be wordless. And it must be because of the fact that Mr. Gurdjieff clearly emphasized how to begin such an investigation. He emphasized that we need first to become whole.

That at least gives us the focus of his exploration. Because according to the great traditions, we are created in the image of God. We are, as it were, three-brained. And Gurdjieff put it very clearly that we need to gather our thoughts. And one does that through these brains. Who am I? Where am I? Am I connected? Do I occupy the body? And do I have this feeling that I need, indeed, to be conscious? Mr. Gurdjieff has given so many indications of how to enter into this investigation. And it all, as it were, comes to a head in Mr. Gurdjieff's own central focus: that life is real only then, when *I Am*. And it is this understanding that nullifies all of the subjectivity with which I face these issues. Because again, Mr. Gurdjieff emphasizes and gives the focus that the central thesis of the teaching is "I Am." And one sees for oneself, as one enters into this wordless inquiry, that "I Am" enters into my vision. It's nothing that I try to describe, innerly, while at the same time trying to grasp the meaning. But even as I sit here now, I have this inkling of the existence of this central force as it begins to penetrate, and as I begin to harken to the resonance in me of "I Am." Madame points out that when I have this opening to that actuality, I am opening—I am opening to Presence. And this opening can't really take place if I am not whole, if it's just my thought or just a tension or sensation in the body that indicates this inner actuality.

So right here at the very doorstep, I am exposed to very central elements in one's being. Indeed it enhances this work to grow in being. Which is no cheap thing. Indeed as I've mentioned many times, Mr. Gurdjieff didn't settle for crumbs. As he'd said to that Christmas gathering here in 1948, he told people to work in a special way—to "Become Christ." And he added: "Be." He didn't say, "Become like Christ," he said, "Become Christ." Which in our understanding is the Son of God, not some makeshift claimant.

Forgive me for struggling to put these thoughts out as I have in the past. This group is a very special one in the way we have focused on the centrality of *I Am* as the pivotal, sustaining force in creation. And so, wordlessly, I enter into this investigation. And when I have the sense of the resonance in me of *I Am*, I am really in touch with the soul. Yet another great mystery.

And so, without any unnecessary or other form of inner talking, I try to investigate this, wordlessly. To occupy the whole. To be in touch with a mind which can be still, and which when it finds itself in the presence of the Creator can acknowledge this reality. This is an extraordinary teaching. Mr. Gurdjieff, as it were, thrusts us in front of this need to serve. We've been created to serve a very high purpose. And one sees one can only fathom its significance in silence, in an inner silence.

And of course it is a big struggle, because ordinarily we are simply slaves of this automaton, which almost ceaselessly affirms itself, and I in turn automatically in my sleep declare that these mechanical affirmations are "I." It is not so. It is not so because all of those automatic affirmations are simply intimations of the ego. And as I've pointed out to you several times, what is real, the real I, is void of the ego. I didn't invent that, it is something Madame put to me one day as I spoke about my effort. It's not an invention, it's not imagination, it has to do with the Real world. And it is that that we're invited to enter when we come together like this. I'm not out to get anything or to flaunt anything, but I am here to serve.

I come here to serve that which is real, and which can only be known through the silence, through what I ordinarily call emptiness. But even the Dalai Lama recently said, extraordinarily, that "Emptiness is consciousness." And we see how much this is lacking and how much it is needed in the world today. As I tried to suggest in the toast on the 13th, even Mother Earth is under siege. And if there is a time that real conscious endeavors are needed, this has the feel of it. Which is a better form of service than all one's hasnamussian endeavors.

Again, this is not an invention. As Madame points out, I am already the being that I would wish to be. But I need to differentiate between the actualities that I serve. This actuality, this transcendent nature, can't be satisfied by the manifestations of what Madame calls one's ferocious egoism. So this is an extraordinary inner encounter that we undertake. And we wish not to be fooled by our inner talk and imagination. So I try to be fully related innerly. And for that I need space, I need to be totally sincere in me, not to be fooled. And I need to respect that my neighbor has this inner life, too. That he or she respects it. And we need to work knowing, as Madame put it, there is no time, only the present moment. This is such an exacting investigation.

And I think it's useful to be reminded, as I was and my colleagues who were in the house the evening when Madame Ouspensky died, way back in Mendham. Two or three days later we received a very touching, respectful letter from Madame de Salzmann in which she spoke reverently of Madame Ouspensky. And right there in the middle of the letter, she said how she was reminded that "There is no death. Life cannot die."

So we have an extraordinary being duty which is to keep this life alive amidst all the threats and the misunderstandings. And so can we bear this in mind, in ourselves, and respect the work, this work to be. Let's work to grow in being. And so can we remember that when we move, when we go into manifestation? `And thank you again for entering into this effort--to keep this connection.

# Part III: The Planet Itself Is Under Pressure

*I used my toast to Mr. Gurdjieff at the 2020 January 13th celebration in New York to sound some dire warnings. This is what I risked saying.*

As we try to contemplate the nature of things—and what better environment than the Foundation in which to make the effort—we need to be reminded, as Madame de Salzmann expressed it so pointedly—that there is no time, only the present moment.

That reminder is ever so relevant when one endeavors to bring a toast for Mr. Gurdjieff, that extraordinary occupant of the present moment.

The Gurdjieff Work is truly an extraordinary teaching. We would indeed have to be clueless, irresponsible, uncaring, mechanical nonentities not to recognize the encompassing effort that is indicated in Madame de Salzmann's penetrating directive: "We must die to the known in order for the unknown to be revealed."

We must die to the known.

Perhaps for most of us it may be true that we have only some (let us say) well-beloved, subjective and egotistic personal priorities. But they are really only further undeniable evidence that we are slaves—again, this is Madame's word—slaves of our automatisms and our voracious egotisms. This in spite of the fact that each of us is created in the image of God—and as Gurdjieff and Madame alert us, there is a cosmic need for the being that I would wish to be.

I will not belabor the point, but there is a need—a cosmic need—to stand in the presence of God and to work for Being. I discover in moments that I am IN God, and that God is IN me. When I learn to listen to the resonance in me of *I Am*, I receive more than an inkling, as the readings have indicated, that we have been created to serve a very great purpose.

But now permit me a little departure from the norm, as I was permitted at the last 13th celebration.

Because there is so much evidence that we are witnessing a significant transformation in our planetary abode. It is the planet, Mother Earth itself, that is under pressure. Just note the surrounding global warming, the threats to many species, the disappearance of entire rain forests—and the hasnamussian antics taking place out in the world.

It is all an extraordinary call to us to wake up to what is Actual, to what is Transcendent, and to what is Real.

So please join me in a toast to this extraordinary man—Mr. Gurdjieff.

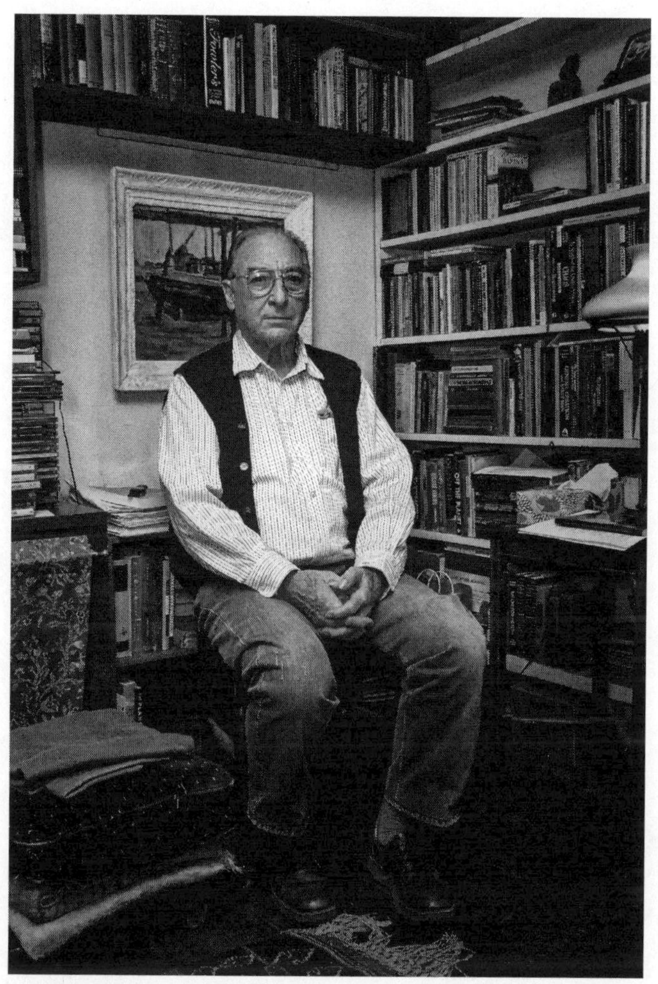

The author.